RENEWED:

Reclaiming Wholeness Through Faith, Health, and Hormone Harmony

By:

K.F. Henry

Cover design by Sylika J. Camacho-Irshad

Forward

I first met Kaleena at church, where we share a strong commitment to community outreach and uplifting our local neighborhood. We quickly connected over our shared backgrounds in healthcare and our passion for improving outcomes for all patients. We also found common ground in mentoring young people, especially those from underserved communities, to pursue meaningful careers in healthcare. We both know that when patients feel a connection rooted in shared experience and community, they are more likely to feel heard, valued, and empowered in their health journeys.

With nearly 20 years of clinical experience, Kaleena brings a rare blend of scientific rigor and real-world wisdom. She has walked alongside patients through setbacks, guided them through complex decisions, and helped them chart sustainable paths toward better health. Her expertise is grounded not just in research, but in compassion—and it shows in the lives she's touched.

This book combines evidence-based insights, biblical principles, and practical strategies for anyone ready to make meaningful, lasting changes in their health. What makes it stand out is Kaleena's ability to translate complex medical concepts into clear, relatable, and actionable advice. You'll feel like you're being guided by someone who not only knows her stuff but genuinely cares about your well-being.

This book couldn't come at a better time. As more women take charge of their health, many are overwhelmed by conflicting information online. Kaleena cuts through the noise, offering trustworthy guidance drawn from clinical experience, credible sources, and most importantly, from scripture. She distills what truly matters and gives you steps you can take today.

Dear reader, I wish you joy, peace, and purpose as you embark on your health journey. With Kaleena's insight and encouragement, you are in excellent hands and on the right path.

Take care,

Tracy MacIntosh, MD MPH MS

Introduction

Faith, Femininity & Flourishing in Every Season

Precious Reader,

You are Seen and Heard.

You are not imagining it.

The fatigue that clings to your bones.
The weight that won't budge—no matter how clean you eat.
The irregular cycles. The blood pressure that spikes.
The mood swings that make you feel like a stranger in your own skin.
The moments when you whisper prayers but wonder why your body still feels like it's falling apart.

You are not broken.
You are not failing.
You are not alone.

This book was written for *you*.

For the Black Christian woman who's trying to stay strong, hold her family together, show up for her church community, and still make sense of the symptoms that never seem to stop.

It's for the woman whose healthcare provider told her "it's just stress" when her hair started falling out.
For the woman who laid hands on her womb, prayed through hot flashes, or fasted through blood sugar crashes.

For the woman who loves Jesus and knows Scripture... but still has questions her provider can't—or won't—answer.

Why This Book Exists

Too often, health books treat our bodies like machines.
Too often, churches over spiritualize what medical wisdom can cure.
And too often, Black women are expected to be strong without ever being supported.

This book is here to break that cycle.

Here, your body is not a problem. It's a temple.
Your hormones are not shameful—they're sacred rhythms.
Your questions are not too big for God—or good medicine.

This book takes a holistic, faith-integrated approach to the *top health challenges affecting Black women*— from hypertension and fibroids to obesity, mental health, PCOS, stroke, and beyond. Through every chapter, we'll explore how hormones, trauma, culture, food, and faith intersect in your story—and how healing is possible at every layer.

A Word of Grace

You will not find shame in these pages.
You will not be told to "just lose weight" or "just have faith."

You will find science, Scripture, and strategies—wrapped in grace.

Because healing isn't just about lab results—it's about liberation.
And wellness isn't just physical—it's emotional, hormonal, generational, and spiritual.

Echoes of Real Women

Throughout these pages, you'll hear the voices of women who have whispered prayers through pain, fasted through fatigue, and fought to reclaim their health – body and soul. Their words come from real stories, interviews, community forums, support groups, and sacred conversations. Their journeys are authentic. Their struggles are familiar. Their courage is holy.

For privacy, names and details have been changed – but the truth of their experiences remains. Each quote is a window into the sacred resilience, spoken in their own way, from their own walk.

These are not fictional fragments. They are echoes of real women.

And in their voices may you hear your own.

You Are Invited

This is more than a book. It's a call to reclaim your health as an act of worship.

To learn. To unlearn. To rise. To rest. To become rooted. To be *whole*.

So let's begin—together.

Let's listen to your body.
Let's seek God for strategy.
Let's reclaim your hormones, your health, and your hope.

Let's write a new story—not just for you, but for your daughters, your sisters, your church, and your legacy.

Because you are not just surviving.
You were made to flourish.

In truth, tenderness, and power,

Kaleena Fransois Henry

Table of Contents

Part I: Understanding the Journey

.

Chapter 1: Menopause – Embracing the Sacred Transition

"Why is no one talking about this? I'm going through menopause, but it feels like I'm all alone in this struggle." – "Keisha," 41, hospitality team leader

"I thought menopause was just hot flashes and mood swings, but my body and mind feel so much more out of control." – "Monica," 47, women's ministry director

---

Menopause: a natural, universal passage that every woman will face. But for Black Christian women, this transition often feels anything but simple or sacred. Menopause means going twelve months without a menstrual cycle, marking the close of one season of life and the opening of another.

Yet, why does it often feel like menopause is the *number one silent struggle* in our churches?

The answer is layered—rooted in silence, misinformation, cultural stigma, and inadequate care. Many women have learned about menopause not through doctors or trusted guides but by watching relatives suffer in quiet or absorbing half-truths from oral traditions, TV, and social media. The reality is, many Black women enter menopause earlier, experience more severe symptoms, and endure longer-lasting effects, yet receive little intentional support.

Common Symptoms You May Recognize

You've probably heard of hot flashes and night sweats—but menopause can show up in many ways, including:

- Sudden warmth, sweating, and flushing (hot flashes)

- Sleepless nights due to night sweats

- Irregular or unpredictable periods before they stop

- Vaginal dryness and discomfort

- Mood swings, irritability, and anxiety

- Fatigue that won't lift

- Weight gain, especially around the belly

- Thinning hair and skin changes

- Difficulty concentrating or "brain fog"

- Joint aches and heart palpitations

- Digestive issues and urinary changes

- Feelings of depression or anxiety

Some women even experience *atypical* symptoms like electric shock sensations, burning skin, tinnitus (ringing in the ears), or anxiety attacks. Symptoms can start years before the last period, often without menopause being part of the conversation with healthcare providers.

You don't need to have every symptom for menopause to matter. Even one can signal a shift requiring care.

Understanding Hormones and Menopause: The Divine Design of Your Body's Messengers

Before we dive deeper into menopause, it's important to understand the powerful hormones that shape your womanhood and health—and how their shifting levels bring about the changes you feel.

Hormones are like God's messengers, sent through your bloodstream to deliver instructions that regulate everything from your mood and energy to your heart health and fertility. Three key hormones take center stage during menopause:

Estrogen
Often called the "queen hormone," estrogen governs many of your body's functions: it keeps your bones strong, your blood vessels flexible, your skin supple, and your moods balanced. Estrogen also regulates your menstrual cycle and helps keep your heart and

brain healthy. During the years leading up to menopause, estrogen levels fluctuate—sometimes wildly—before eventually declining steadily after your last period.

Progesterone

Progesterone works alongside estrogen, preparing your body for potential pregnancy each month. It also helps regulate mood and supports restful sleep. Like estrogen, progesterone levels begin to drop during perimenopause, contributing to symptoms like irregular periods and mood swings.

Other Hormones

- **Testosterone** — yes, women have it too! It supports libido, energy, and muscle strength but also declines with age.

- **Follicle-Stimulating Hormone (FSH)** and **Luteinizing Hormone (LH)** — these signal your ovaries to produce estrogen and progesterone. As your ovaries slow down, these hormone levels rise as the body tries to stimulate hormone production.

- **Cortisol** — the stress hormone, which often rises during menopause due to physical and emotional stress, worsening symptoms.

What Happens During Menopause?

As the ovaries produce less estrogen and progesterone, your body feels the ripple effects:

- Blood vessels lose flexibility, leading to hot flashes and increased risk of high blood pressure and heart disease.

- Bone density decreases, raising the risk for osteoporosis.

- The brain's neurotransmitter balance shifts, contributing to mood swings, anxiety, and memory fog.

- Metabolism slows, making weight gain easier and weight loss harder.

- Vaginal tissues thin and dry, causing discomfort and increasing infection risks.

These changes are natural but can feel overwhelming—especially when symptoms arrive suddenly or persist longer than expected.

Why Menopause Matters So Deeply

Menopause doesn't just change your cycles—it impacts your whole body and intersects with many health challenges that disproportionately affect Black women, including:

- **Heart disease:** Estrogen protects the heart and blood vessels; its loss raises risks of hypertension, stroke, and heart attacks.

- **Diabetes:** Hormonal shifts can worsen insulin resistance, increasing diabetes risk.

- **Obesity:** Metabolic rate slows, fat redistributes, and weight gain often follows.

- **Breast cancer:** Hormonal changes influence breast tissue; fat tissue after menopause can produce estrogen linked to certain cancers.

- **Mental health:** Mood swings, anxiety, and depression often intensify.

- **Autoimmune diseases:** Conditions like lupus may worsen with hormonal changes.

- **Other concerns:** Increased risk of osteoporosis, asthma exacerbations, vaginal atrophy increasing infection risks.

For many Black women, these risks are compounded by systemic health disparities, stress, and lack of culturally sensitive care.

Faith and the Journey Through Menopause

Menopause can feel like a spiritual battle as much as a physical one.

- *"I pray for peace, but the night sweats and mood swings don't stop."*

- *"Am I losing my womanhood? My strength? Is this God's plan for me?"*

- *"Why does this transition feel so isolating when the church doesn't talk about it?"*

Remember: God created every season of life with purpose. Your body's changes are not punishment or failure. The Psalmist reminds us:

> "For everything there is a season, and a time for every matter under heaven."
> — Ecclesiastes 3:1 (ESV)

And Jesus walks with us in every season—not just the easy ones.

Wholeness Strategy: Embracing Menopause with Faith and Function

Medical & Hormonal Support

- Talk openly with your healthcare provider about symptoms. Request hormone panels or pelvic ultrasounds if needed.

- Consider safe, evidence-based treatments like bioidentical hormone therapy (BHT) or non-hormonal medications to ease symptoms. BHT is the preferred option because it uses hormones that are molecularly identical to the ones your body naturally produces, such as estradiol and progesterone. Because they closely mimic your body's own hormones, bioidentical hormones can offer symptom relief more precisely than non-hormone options with potentially fewer side effects compared to synthetic hormone therapies. This personalized approach aims to restore hormonal balance gently and safely, tailored to your unique needs.

- Understand risks and benefits, especially around hormone replacement therapy, and ask questions about personalized care.

Nutritional Healing

- Include *phytoestrogen-rich* foods like soy, flaxseed, and lentils to support estrogen balance.

- Choose calcium and vitamin D-rich foods for bone health: leafy greens, fortified milks, fatty fish.

- Favor fiber, lean proteins, and healthy fats to support metabolism and weight.

- Avoid triggers like spicy foods, caffeine, alcohol, and highly processed foods that worsen symptoms.

Lifestyle Shifts

- Prioritize restful sleep; create soothing bedtime routines and manage night sweats with breathable bedding.

- Engage in gentle exercise like walking, yoga, or dancing to boost mood and metabolism.

- Practice stress-reduction techniques: prayer, breathwork, meditation, and Sabbath rest.

Spiritual Anchors

- *"The LORD is near to the brokenhearted and saves the crushed in spirit."* — Psalm 34:18 (ESV)

- *"Come to me, all who labor and are heavy laden, and I will give you rest."* — Matthew 11:28 (ESV)

- *"She is clothed with strength and dignity; she can laugh at the days to come."* — Proverbs 31:25 (NIV)

- **Journal Prompt:** *"What fears or frustrations about menopause am I holding onto? How can I invite God's peace into those places today?"*

- **Prayer:**
  Lord, guide me through this season of change. Help me honor the body You've given me and find strength in Your presence. Teach me to walk in grace and wisdom as I embrace this sacred transition.

Voices of Encouragement

"I used to think menopause was a curse, but now I see it as a new chapter God wrote for me." – "Aunt Glo," 63, Georgia

"Finding a provider who respects my faith and listens to my story changed everything." – A.C, 44, worship leader

"My symptoms don't define me—God's love does." – T.J., 51, Bible study leader

---

Menopause is a journey—sometimes challenging, often misunderstood—but always sacred. It is not the end, but a beginning: a time to renew, restore, and reclaim your wholeness in body, mind, and spirit.

You are fearfully and wonderfully made, in every season of life (Psalm 139:14).

Let this chapter be the first step in speaking openly, caring deeply, and walking boldly into your next season with faith, hope, and healing.

Chapter 2: The Pressures Within – Finding Peace Amid High Blood Pressure

---

"I'm doing everything right—cutting back on salt, walking every day, praying for peace—and my blood pressure is still high. What more can I do?" – T.L., retired teacher, Florida

---

You've probably heard the term "high blood pressure," or maybe the more clinical name: hypertension. It sounds simple enough—just a number on a cuff, right?

But for Black Christian women, it's far more than that.

Hypertension is often called the *silent killer* because it rarely announces itself with obvious symptoms. Yet behind the scenes, it's hard at work—damaging your heart, straining your kidneys, fogging your brain, and slowly draining your strength.

And it's not rare. In fact, nearly **1 in 2 Black women** in the U.S. lives with hypertension, often undiagnosed or untreated. That means if you look around your church pew on Sunday, it's likely that half the women worshipping beside you are carrying this silent load too.

Understanding the Numbers

Let's break down what high blood pressure actually means:

- **Normal:** Less than **120/80 mmHg**

- **Elevated: 120-129** systolic (top number) and **less than 80** diastolic (bottom number)

- **Stage 1 Hypertension: 130-139** systolic or **80-89** diastolic

- **Stage 2 Hypertension: 140 or higher** systolic or **90 or higher** diastolic

- **Hypertensive Crisis: 180+/120+** — this requires immediate medical attention.

These numbers matter because even a small elevation—consistently above 130/80—can lead to major health problems over time.

The Real Dangers of Hypertension

If left untreated, high blood pressure can result in:

- **Heart disease:** It forces your heart to work harder, increasing the risk of heart attacks, heart failure, and arrhythmias.

- **Stroke:** It damages and narrows arteries, increasing the chance of blood clots and strokes.

- **Kidney failure:** High pressure can weaken the blood vessels in your kidneys, leading to decreased function or dialysis.

- **Vision loss:** Yes—hypertension can damage the tiny vessels in your eyes.

- **Cognitive decline:** Studies now link high blood pressure with dementia and memory loss.

But here's what often gets missed in the conversation: Black women don't just have higher rates—we tend to have more severe outcomes, and we often develop these conditions earlier in life.

Why?

Because our bodies aren't just responding to sodium and stress. They're responding to years of compounded emotional trauma, racial microaggressions, economic stressors, and the invisible pressure to be strong for everyone else.

"They told me to relax. I wanted to scream. I've been holding it down for my family, my church, my community—and now they want me to pretend like peace is a bubble bath?" – "Ebony," 40, single mom and choir assistant

The Hormone Connection

Here's a truth the average doctor doesn't explain: as we approach our 40s and beyond, our hormone levels begin shifting—and those shifts can spike our blood pressure in sneaky ways.

- **Estrogen**, which helps blood vessels stay relaxed and flexible, starts to decline during perimenopause and drops sharply after menopause.

- **Cortisol**, your stress hormone, can skyrocket from chronic pressure or even poor sleep— both common in midlife women.

- **Insulin resistance**, which increases with age and hormonal shifts, can contribute to vascular damage.

When these hormones go out of balance, your blood pressure isn't just reacting to what you ate—it's reacting to what you feel, how you sleep, how you breathe, and what your body is trying to survive.

"My body feels like it's stuck in survival mode—even when I'm resting." – D.C., 41, registered nurse

Faith Under Pressure

For women of faith, there's often an added layer of guilt.

"I pray for peace, but the tension stays in my shoulders." – "Shonda," 48, Georgia

"I'm tired of asking God for healing when my numbers never go down." – "Tamika," 44, Alabama

"I feel like I'm failing—spiritually and physically." –
J.M., 38, praise team leader

But here's the truth: prayer is powerful, but it's not a substitute for medical care or understanding your body. Scripture doesn't pit faith against wisdom—it marries them.

"The heart of the discerning acquires knowledge, for the ears of the wise seek it out." — Proverbs 18:15 (NIV)

Seeking healing in your body isn't unspiritual—it's biblical. You are not weak for needing help. You are not broken for needing medicine. You are a daughter of God in need of both *grace* and *strategy*.

Wholeness Strategy: Faith Meets Function

Let's move from awareness to action. Healing starts with understanding, but it's sustained by choices—small, sacred, and steady ones.

Medical & Hormonal Support

- **Get tested:** Ask your provider for a full hormone panel and a home BP monitor.

- **Don't delay meds:** If you're prescribed blood pressure medication, take it as instructed.

- **Ask questions:** Seek a provider who listens to your story—not just your numbers.

Nutritional Healing

- **DASH-style eating:** Focus on potassium-rich foods (spinach, sweet potatoes, avocados), whole grains, beans, and lean protein.

- **Flavor swaps:** Use herbs, lemon, and garlic instead of salt.

- **Sugar check:** Cut back on hidden sugars that increase inflammation.

What Is DASH-Style Eating?

When I say "DASH-style," I'm not talking about another trendy diet. DASH stands for Dietary Approaches to Stop Hypertension – and it's one of the most research-backed eating plans for lowering blood pressure naturally.

But more than that – it's about eating in a way that nourishes your heart, honors your culture, and supports your temple.

A DASH-style approach focuses on:

- **Plenty of fruits and vegetables** (especially leafy greens, berries, sweet potatoes)
- **Whole grains** (like brown rice, quinoa, oats, whole grain grits)
- **Low-fat or non-dairy alternatives**
- **Heart-healthy fats** (olive oil, avocado, nuts, seeds)
- **Herbs and spices instead of salt** (like garlic, thyme, lemon, and smoked paprika)

And it means *reducing things like:*

- Sodium (from canned goods, fast food, seasoning blends)
- Sugary drinks and sweets
- Fried and highly processed foods
- Red meat and high-fat dairy

Think: greens with smoked turkey instead of ham hocks. Roasted sweet potatoes instead of fries. A cup of fruit-infused water instead of soda.

This isn't about perfection – it's about protection. Protection for your heart, kidneys, your brain, and your future. Even small changes, made consistently, can lead to big healing.

Lifestyle Shifts

- **Holy walking:** 20–30 minutes of daily walking with prayer or worship music.

- **Sabbath rest:** Weekly intentional rest—no guilt, no striving.

- **Breathwork:** Try 4-7-8 breathing (*inhale* through your nose for *4 seconds*, *hold* your breath for *7 seconds*, and *exhale* slowly through your mouth for *8 seconds*) before bed to lower cortisol and promote peace.

Spiritual Anchors

- **Philippians 4:6-7 (KJV):** *"Be careful for nothing... and the peace of God... shall keep your hearts and minds."*

- **Proverbs 4:23 (NASB):** *"Watch over your heart with all diligence..."*

- **Journal Prompt:** "Where is pressure weighing heavier than grace in my life?"

- **Daily Breath Prayer:** *"Be still... and know that I am God."*

Voices of Wisdom

"Once I stopped performing and started protecting my peace, my BP started dropping." - K.S., 35, choir member, Maryland

"I realized I wasn't just saving my life—I was breaking a generational curse." - "Cherelle," 57, youth leader and caregiver

"I don't need to be everyone's everything. That's God's job. Mine is to breathe." – M.R., 27, Mississippi

---

You were never meant to carry this pressure alone. And the solution isn't just pills or kale smoothies—it's reclaiming your body as holy ground, created and loved by a God who sees every part of your struggle.

This is the beginning of renewal. Not just lower numbers—but higher peace.

Chapter 3: Blood Sugar Battles – Finding Balance with Faith and Physiology

---

"I just found out I'm prediabetic. I'm scared—but also so tired of trying to fix my body when nothing seems to work." – "Jennifer," 41, mother of three

"My mother lost her legs to diabetes. I don't want that to be my story too." – A.B., 38, youth mentor

---

When it comes to blood sugar issues—prediabetes, insulin resistance, and type 2 diabetes—many Black Christian women are caught between fear, frustration, and fatigue. And for good reason: diabetes is one of the top health challenges we face.

But the story doesn't have to end in panic or hopelessness. Understanding your hormones, your habits, and your heritage can open the door to real, sustainable healing—body and soul.

The Weight of the Numbers

Let's get real about what the numbers mean:

- **Normal fasting blood sugar:** Less than **100 mg/dL**

- **Prediabetes: 100–125 mg/dL**

- **Type 2 Diabetes: 126 mg/dL or higher** on two separate tests

- **A1C (3-month blood sugar average):**

    o Normal: **below 5.7%**

    o Prediabetes: **5.7–6.4%**

    o Diabetes: **6.5% or higher**

The problem is, many of us walk around with elevated blood sugar for years before getting diagnosed. Why? Because we've been told it's normal to feel tired, to crave sugar, to have belly weight that won't budge. But normal doesn't mean healthy.

Tools to Track and Transform

If you want to get ahead of your numbers, **know your patterns**:

- A **glucometer** is a small device that uses a drop of blood from your finger to check your current blood sugar level. It's simple, affordable, and great for spot-checks—especially before and after meals.

- A **Continuous Glucose Monitor (CGM)** is a sensor worn on your skin (usually your arm or abdomen) that tracks your blood sugar throughout the day and night—without finger pricks. You can see how your body responds to specific meals, stress, or sleep. This tool is especially empowering because it gives **real-time feedback** to help you course-correct quickly.

If you've ever wondered, *"Why am I so tired after lunch?"* or *"Is this snack causing a crash?"*—a CGM can reveal the truth and guide your healing.

Hormones and the Sugar Spiral

Blood sugar issues are more than just what you eat—they're how your **hormones** are working behind the scenes.

- **Insulin** helps your cells absorb glucose (sugar). If you're resistant to insulin, sugar stays in your bloodstream, leading to weight gain, fatigue, and eventually diabetes.

- **Cortisol**, the stress hormone, increases blood sugar when you're overwhelmed—even without food.

- **Estrogen and progesterone**, especially during perimenopause and menopause, influence how your body stores fat and manages sugar.

That's why some women say:

"I was eating the same as I always have—but now I'm gaining weight, and my labs are off." – K.S., 47, business owner

Here's what most women are never told:

Your menstrual cycle also affects your insulin sensitivity.

During the follicular phase (the first half of your cycle, from menstruation to ovulation), insulin sensitivity is typically higher. This means your body processes carbohydrates more efficiently, and your energy levels may be more stable. It's often the ideal time for highter-intensity workouts or adjusting carb intake without major blood sugar crashes.

During the luteal phase (the second half of your cycle, after ovulation), progesterone rises and insulin sensitivity decreases. As a result, your body may become more pronte to blood sugar spkes and cravings – especially for sweets and carbs. You may feel more tired, foggy, or emotionally sensitive, which can lead to reactive eating.

This isn't weakness – it's wisdom your body is offering.

Your hormones shifted. And no one told you how to adjust. When your body stores belly fat, craves sugar, or crashes after meals, it's speaking. Let's take the time to learn to listen. When you learn to eat and live in rhythm with your cycle, you can reduce the burden on your metabolism and create space for healing. "There is a time for everything... a season for every activity under the heavens." – Ecclesiastes 3:1 (NIV)

Your body follows a divine rhythm. When you honor
it, you walk in wisdom – not restriction.

Blood Sugar & Hormone Support Through the Menstrual Cycle

Here's a practical breakdown of how each phase impacts blood sugar and how you
can support your body with grace and intention:

1. Menstrual Phase (Days 1–5)
Hormones: Estrogen and progesterone are at their lowest.
Insulin Sensitivity: Moderate to high.
What You May Feel: Fatigue, cramps, emotional sensitivity.
Support Strategy: Eat iron-rich foods like leafy greens, lentils, and beets. Focus on
warm, nourishing meals. Gentle movement like stretching or prayer walks. Prioritize
rest and reflection.

2. Follicular Phase (Days 6–14)
Hormones: Estrogen rises; progesterone remains low.
Insulin Sensitivity: Highest during this time.
What You May Feel: Increased energy, mental clarity, light appetite.
Support Strategy: Best time for complex carbs like quinoa, oats, and fruits.
Incorporate strength training or higher-intensity movement. Plan meals and
routines—your brain is sharpest now. Use this window to build healthy habits.

3. Ovulation (Days 14–16)
Hormones: Estrogen peaks; luteinizing hormone (LH) surges.
Insulin Sensitivity: Still fairly high.
What You May Feel: Sociable, energetic, slightly hungrier.
Support Strategy: Focus on balanced meals with protein, fat, and fiber. Stay hydrated
and stabilize energy with frequent, small meals. Great time for community activities
or church involvement. Watch out for skipped meals—your energy can mask hunger.

4. Luteal Phase (Days 15–28)
Hormones: Progesterone rises, estrogen begins to fall.
Insulin Sensitivity: Decreases—more prone to blood sugar spikes.
What You May Feel: Bloating, cravings (especially sweets), mood swings, fatigue.
Support Strategy: Choose low-glycemic carbs like sweet potatoes and lentils. Add
magnesium-rich foods (dark chocolate, pumpkin seeds). Honor cravings with
healthier swaps (fruit + nuts). Prioritize rest, spiritual grounding, and boundaries.

Note: Cycle lengths vary. These are average ranges based on a 28-day cycle.

Your body isn't unpredictable—it's divinely designed.
By honoring your hormone rhythm, you can reduce inflammation, stabilize
your blood sugar, and find peace in your process.

Faith and Food: The Battle Within

So many of us have a complicated relationship with food. We eat when we're stressed. We eat to celebrate. We eat what's familiar—even when it hurts us.

And in the church? It gets harder.

"Church potlucks are my downfall—how do I honor God with my plate when greens are cooked in pork?"
- C.L.,66, church hospitality coordinator

"Fasting left me dizzy — but I didn't want to seem weak in front of my sisters." – "Tasha," 39, Florida

We are often encouraged to "pray over our portions" or fast more—but very few of us are taught how to support our bodies after the prayer or during the fast. Fasting is a beautiful spiritual discipline. But without proper knowledge, it can backfire—especially for women with blood sugar issues.

Here's how to support your body during or after a fast:

- **Hydration:** Start your fast with water infused with lemon or cucumber, and sip throughout to support blood sugar and flush toxins.

- **Break your fast with balance:** Choose a meal with protein, healthy fat, and fiber to avoid a blood sugar spike. Example: Grilled chicken, sautéed greens, and quinoa.

- **During a fast (if extended):** Consider adding herbal teas (like cinnamon or ginger) and mineral-rich bone broth to stabilize energy.

- **After prayer time:** Instead of reaching for a quick carb (like muffins or juice), try nuts, boiled eggs, or hummus with veggies—these nourish without triggering a glucose surge.

This isn't about willpower — it's about wisdom.

Scripture says, *"Whether you eat or drink, or whatever you do, do all to the glory of God."* (1 Corinthians 10:31, NASB)

That includes making peace with food—not as an enemy or idol—but as fuel to fulfill your purpose.

The Damaging Effects of Diabetes

If left unchecked, diabetes doesn't just stay in the bloodstream. It attacks your entire body:

- **Heart disease and stroke**

- **Kidney damage (leading to dialysis)**

- **Nerve damage (causing pain or numbness)**

- **Eye damage and vision loss**

- **Slow healing and infections**

- **Emotional strain, depression, and shame**

For Black women, complications often set in faster due to later diagnoses and less access to culturally competent care.

"By the time they told me I had diabetes, I already had neuropathy. No one explained what was happening before that." – V.S., 64, Georgia

You deserve better.

Wholeness Strategy: Resetting the Temple

Healing starts with grace. Not guilt. Not crash diets. Not miracle shakes.

Just grace.

Medical & Hormonal Support

- Ask for **A1C, fasting insulin, and thyroid markers**—not just glucose.

- If your provider recommends prescriptions like **metformin** or a **GLP-1 agonist** (like Ozempic or Mounjaro), don't let fear block your healing. These aren't signs of failure – they're tools. Metformin helps your cells respond better to insulin. GLP-1s reduce appetite, calm inflammation, support insulin balance, and protect the kidneys and the heart. Used together or independently, can be very effective, especially if you're trying to reverse early insulin resistance. When used wisely, they can give your body the *breathing room* it needs to optimize functioning.

- Ask about using a **CGM** for a more personalized understanding of your body's responses.

- Consider a hormone tracking device like **Mira** (can be purchased at www.MiraCare.com without a prescription). It monitors specific hormones like estrogen, progesterone, LH, and FSH in real-time. This can be used for various purposes, including fertility tracking, perimenopause monitoring, or understanding overall hormonal health. It's a great way to learn about your individual cycle rhythm.

Nutritional Healing

- Eat in harmony with your hormones:

    o Protein + fiber at every meal

    o Healthy fats (avocado, olive oil, nuts)

    o Whole, colorful foods—not processed sugars

- Watch your portions, not just your prayers.

    o Use a smaller plate to naturally eat less.

    o Eat slowly, allowing your body to signal fullness.

- Measuring trigger foods (like rice or bread) instead of eyeballing.

- Honoring hunger – not guilt – when making decisions.

Protein + Fiber = Blood Sugar Allies

Pairing **protein** and **fiber** helps slow down digestion and stabilize blood sugar.

- **Protein examples:** Eggs, turkey, chicken, Greek yogurt, lentils, tofu, fish, or beans.

- **Fiber examples:** Leafy greens, chia seeds, broccoli, apples (with skin), flaxseed, oats, and legumes.

Think: a spinach salad with grilled salmon and a sprinkle of pumpkin seeds. Or oatmeal with a scoop of protein powder and berries.

These combinations prevent energy crashes and support hormone balance.

- Simple modifications with big impact:

  - Swap sugary breakfast cereals for savory veggie omelets or steel-cut oats with cinnamon.

  - Embrace sweet alternatives: cinnamon, berries, stevia, and balanced carbs like sweet potatoes.

  - Cook collards with smoked turkey instead of ham hocks.

  - Prep "grab-and-go" snacks that combine protein and fiber: almonds + apple, boiled eggs + cherry tomatoes.

Lifestyle Shifts

- Move daily—not for weight loss, but for blood sugar control (even 10 minutes after meals can significantly lower blood sugar spikes).

- Prioritize consistent sleep—lack of rest raises cortisol and blood sugar.

- Manage stress with Scripture, silence, and support.

Spiritual Anchors

- **Galatians 5:22-23 (NIV):** *"The fruit of the Spirit is... self-control."*

- **Romans 12:1 (NASB):** *"Present your bodies as a living and holy sacrifice, acceptable to God..."*

- **Journal Prompt:** "How has food become comfort instead of fuel in my life?"

- **Prayer:** "Lord, help me find balance—not bondage—in how I care for this body You gave me. Teach me to treat food as a blessing, not a battleground."

Voices of Victory

"I thought taking medicine meant I wasn't doing enough. But I realized it was a form of grace – God using science to support my healing." – D.C., 32, church member

"I stopped dieting and started learning. Now I eat with peace, not punishment." – "Renee," 50, retail clerk

"Understanding insulin resistance changed everything—it wasn't just about willpower." - M.R., 52, mother and grandmother

"I don't fear food anymore. I fear losing my calling if I don't take care of me." – "Shana," 35, youth leader

---

You are not a sugar addict. Your cravings do not cancel your calling. You're not a failure. You are a woman called to wholeness—and God is with you in every bite, every prayer, and every decision toward balance. With every step—spiritually and physically—you are choosing to be free.

Freedom doesn't come from fear. It comes from truth, grace, and wisdom.

You're not disqualified from healing. So, let's keep walking toward it – one balanced meal, one prayer, one day at a time.

Chapter 4: Heart Disease – Loving the Heart That Loves So Many

---

"I take care of everybody—my kids, my husband, my church—but my heart doesn't feel okay." – "Monica," 48, caregiver and Sunday school leader

"They said it was anxiety. Turned out I'd already had a minor heart attack." – M.J., 41, Georgia

---

Heart disease is the number one killer of women in America. But for Black women, it is particularly dangerous and often undetected until it's too late.

In fact, nearly **50% of Black women over age 20** have some form of cardiovascular disease. And many of them never know it until they're hospitalized—or worse.

"I thought I was just tired. No one told me fatigue could be a heart symptom." – A.B., 48

We're taught to love others, serve faithfully, and keep going no matter what. But what happens when the heart that loves so many starts to wear down?

It's time to listen—to the science, to the Spirit, and to your own heartbeat.

The Real Risks for Real Women

Let's be clear: Black women face a **disproportionately higher risk** for heart disease due to a complex combination of biology, stress, social pressures, hormonal pressures, and systemic disparities.

Risk factors include:

- **High blood pressure**

- **High cholesterol**

- **Diabetes or insulin resistance**

- **Obesity or excess belly fat**

- **Smoking**

- **Chronic stress and poor sleep**

- **Family history of heart disease or stroke**

- **Menopause** – especially after age 45

Yes, menopause belongs on that list. The sharp drop in **estrogen** during and after this transition removes a key layer of protection from your cardiovascular system.

And when your **stress hormones** like cortisol stay elevated—whether from caregiving, racism, grief, or constant striving—it puts your heart under chronic, silent strain.

"I didn't know burnout could break my body." – "Vicky," 47, hair stylist

While these risks are serious, they are not final. Understanding them is the first act of healing.

How Hormones Shape the Heart

Estrogen – your primary female hormone - helps your blood vessels stay open, flexible, and less prone to inflammation. When estrogen declines—especially after menopause—your risk for:

- High blood pressure

- Unhealthy cholesterol

- Arterial plaque buildup

- Insulin resistance and belly fat

...all increases. This means a woman who once had "normal" heart health can become high-risk **in just a few years**, simply because of natural hormonal shifts.

This is not to make you fear menopause—but to help you prepare for it, *wisely and holistically.*

Silent but Serious: How Women Experience Heart Disease

We've been taught to expect chest pain as the classic heart attack symptom. But in women – especially

Black women – heart symptoms can be subtle or misleading. We often experience:

- Shortness of breath (even at rest)
- Unusual or Extreme fatigue (especially after sleep)
- Jaw, back, or arm pain
- Heartburn, nausea, or lightheadedness
- Dizziness, anxiety, or fainting
- Palpitations or a fluttering chest

Don't ignore these signs. If something feels "off," don't dismiss it. Your heart speaks. Learn to listen - and advocate for your heart.

Faith and the Heart's Burden

Scripture speaks often of the heart—guarding it, purifying it, strengthening it. But many women of faith live in constant contradiction: pouring out love for others while neglecting their own beating vessel. We give so much of ourselves in love—sometimes to our own detriment. Unfortunately, we too often equate self-care with selfishness.

"My heart serves everyone else. I just want to know if anyone sees when it's breaking." – K.S., 37, Alabama

But God sees. And He cares. He wants your heart whole — not worn out.

- *"Above all else, guard your heart, for everything you do flows from it."* – Proverbs 4:23 (NIV)

- *"My flesh and my heart may fail, but God is the strength of my heart..."* – Psalm 73:26 (NASB)

God is not asking you to run yourself into the ground in His name. He's asking you to guard the heart He gave you. Let His strength become your standard— not exhaustion.

Wholeness Strategy: Caring for the Heart That Cares for Others

Medical & Hormonal Support

- Schedule routine checks for blood pressure, cholesterol, and A1C—especially post-menopause.

- If you're at higher risk (family history, menopause, high cholesterol, etc.), request a calcium heart scan. This non-invasive test measures plaque buildup in your arteries, revealing hidden risks before a heart attack occurs. It's particularly useful for women whose symptoms are often missed or dismissed.

- If you're postmenopausal, ask your doctor how hormonal changes may be affecting your cardiovascular health. Discuss whether HRT (hormone replacement therapy) is appropriate

for you—especially if heart disease runs in
your family.

Nutritional Healing

- Heart-loving foods include:

    - **Healthy fats**: Olive oil, nuts, avocado,
      salmon

    - **Soluble fiber**: Oats, apples, beans,
      lentils

    - **Anti-inflammatory choices**: Berries,
      dark leafy greens, turmeric

- Minimize: Trans fats, fried foods, sugary
  drinks, added sugars, and excess sodium –
  especially from processed snacks/foods

- Try:

    - Replacing red meat with fatty fish

    - Snacking on walnuts instead of chips

    - Seasoning with herbs and lemon
      instead of salt

- Add heart-supporting nutrients: magnesium
  (leafy greens), potassium (bananas, sweet
  potatoes), and CoQ10 (available as a
  supplement)

Lifestyle Shifts

- **Move with joy**—dancing, walking, water aerobics, or even gardening. 30 minutes a day can transform your heart health.

- Create a wind-down routine to promote restful sleep (at least 7-8 hours) — deep sleep helps to regulate blood and repair/heal your heart.

- Reduce chronic stress through worship, deep breathing, and healthy boundaries —your heart is not a dumping ground for everyone's crisis. Saying "no" is a form of protection.

Spiritual Anchors

- **Psalm 147:3 (NASB):** *"He heals the brokenhearted and binds up their wounds."*

- **Isaiah 26:3 (KJV):** *"Thou wilt keep him in perfect peace, whose mind is stayed on thee..."*

- **Journal Prompt:** "What burdens am I carrying that are breaking my heart in silence? What burdens have I been carrying that are too heavy for my heart?"

- **Breath Prayer:** Inhale – *"Jesus, give me peace."* Exhale – *"Strengthen my heart."*

Voices of Renewal

"I didn't know peace could be a prescription. But once I stopped carrying everyone else's expectations,

my pressure dropped." – "Danielle," 50, retired
teacher, Ohio

*"I found healing when I learned to say 'no' without
guilt and 'yes' to myself."*- L.M., 44, single mother

*"God didn't ask me to die for the church. Jesus
already did that."* – "Monica," 49, first lady

Your heart is not just a pump—it's the wellspring of
your spirit. Your heart is sacred – not because of how
much it can give, but because of Who gave it to you.
It is worth protecting, nourishing, and restoring like
the sacred vessel it is.

Let your healing begin not in fear, but in faith and
informed love. Let your healing be an act of worship.
Let your wholeness be your testimony.

Your heart has given so much. Now it's time to give
back to it. This is your permission to love the heart
that loves so many – starting with your own.

Chapter 5: Body and Image – Overcoming Obesity with Compassion and Care

---

"No matter what I do, the weight won't budge — especially around my belly." – "Tanya," 39, mom of two

"I feel trapped in a body that doesn't reflect who I am inside." - T.M., 51, retired dance instructor

---

Weight. For many of us, it's more than a number on a scale. It's tied to identity, shame, frustration, and fear. It's the silent companion to every doctor's visit, the inner critic at every mirror, and the unspoken pressure during every church function.

And it's complicated.

Because for Black Christian women, obesity isn't just a matter of calories or willpower. It's often the result of hormonal imbalances, generational trauma, food apartheid, and a lifetime of being told to be "strong," even when our bodies are breaking under the weight—literally and emotionally.

The Truth Behind the Numbers

According to the CDC, **about 57% of Black women in the U.S. are classified as obese** — the highest rate among all racial and gender groups. And with obesity comes an increased risk for:

- Type 2 diabetes

- Heart disease

- High blood pressure

- Stroke

- Sleep apnea

- Joint pain

- Certain cancers

- Infertility and PCOS

But those are just the physical risks. The emotional toll is just as heavy:

- Being judged at church or family gatherings

- Feeling invisible or undesirable

- Constant yo-yo dieting that never works long-term

- Internal battles between faith, food, and self-worth

"My self-esteem is suffering, and I'm tired of feeling invisible."- S.P., 35, flight attendant

The Hormone–Weight Connection

If you've ever said, *"I'm doing everything right, but the weight won't move,"* you're not imagining things.

Here's why your hormones matter:

- **Cortisol (stress hormone)**: Constant stress elevates cortisol, which promotes belly fat storage — especially dangerous visceral fat.

- **Insulin**: When cells stop responding properly to insulin (insulin resistance), it becomes easier to gain weight and harder to burn fat.

- **Estrogen and progesterone**: Decline during perimenopause and menopause can slow metabolism and shift fat to the midsection.

- **Thyroid hormones**: Often underdiagnosed in Black women, a sluggish thyroid can reduce metabolism and increase fatigue.

All these imbalances make traditional advice like *"eat less and move more"* overly simplistic and often harmful.

"My thyroid test came back 'normal,' but I'm gaining weight eating salads — what's the secret?!" - K.S., 47, small group leader, South Carolina

The secret? It's not your fault. But it *is* your opportunity to reset — gently, wisely, and with compassion.

Faith, Food, and the Fullness of Life

Food is deeply spiritual. It's communal. It's cultural. It's how we fellowship, how we celebrate, and sometimes, how we cope.

So when we're told to just "eat clean" or "cut carbs," it feels like we're being asked to cut off parts of our story.

"I feel like I'm sinning every time I eat something that tastes good." – "Mikayla," 39, social worker

We need more than just rules. We need redemption— a new way to view our bodies and our plates through the lens of grace.

- *"So whether you eat or drink... do all to the glory of God." –* 1 Corinthians 10:31 (NASB)

- *"You are fearfully and wonderfully made..." –* Psalm 139:14 (KJV)

This isn't about shrinking to fit in. It's about stewarding your body so you can fully show up for the purpose God placed in you.

Wholeness Strategy: Compassionate Weight Management

Medical & Hormonal Support

- Request testing for:

  - **Thyroid function** (TSH, Free T3, Free T4)

  - **Fasting insulin and cortisol**

  - **Vitamin D and B12** (often low in Black women and can impact energy and metabolism)

- Discuss options like **GLP-1 medications** (e.g., Ozempic, Wegovy, Zepbound, Liraglutide) or **metformin** with your provider, especially if insulin resistance is present.

Nutritional Healing

- Focus on **metabolic balance**, not restriction:
    - **Protein**: Eggs, fish, legumes, turkey
    - **Fiber**: Chia seeds, lentils, leafy greens
    - **Healthy fats**: Avocado, olive oil, almonds
- Stabilize your meals:
    - Eat every 4–5 hours to support blood sugar and hormone rhythms.
    - Don't skip meals — it can raise cortisol and slow metabolism.
- Simple adaptations to loved recipes:
    - Swap white rice for cauliflower rice or quinoa.
    - Season greens with smoked turkey or herbs instead of pork.
    - Choose baked, grilled, or air-fried options instead of fried.

Lifestyle Shifts

- Wear a continuous glucose monitor routinely to inform dietary and lifestyle behavioral changes.

- Move joyfully: Dance, walk, stretch — whatever brings delight, not dread.

- Aim for strength and stamina, not just weight loss.

- Sleep like it's sacred: Fat loss and hormone regulation depend on deep rest.

- Stop the comparison trap: Your journey is yours. What works for others may not work for your uniquely blessed body.

Spiritual Anchors

- **Romans 12:1 (KJV):** *"Present your bodies a living sacrifice, holy... unto God."*

- **1 Samuel 16:7 (NIV):** *"The Lord does not look at the things people look at... the Lord looks at the heart."*

- **Journal Prompt:** "How have I equated my worth with my weight?"

- **Prayer:** "Lord, help me love this body You've given me — not when it changes, but as it is. Help me honor You through how I nourish and care for it."

Voices of Courage

"I stopped chasing skinny. I started chasing strength."- "Cherelle," 33, praise dancer

"The weight didn't define me — but my health needed my attention." – B.H., 60, grandmother

"Once I fed my soul with truth, I stopped starving my body with shame." – M.R., 52, cashier, Georgia

---

You don't need to punish your body into submission. You need to partner with it in healing.

You're not called to look a certain way—you're called to live fully, joyfully, and with vitality.

Let your journey toward wholeness begin with compassion — not control.

Chapter 6: Waging War Within – Breast Cancer and the Fight for Hope

---

"I never thought it would be me. No one in my family had breast cancer."- "Tamara," 43, social worker

"They found it late. I kept putting off my mammogram because I was too busy taking care of everyone else." – V.T., 56, registered nurse and caregiver

---

Breast cancer isn't just a medical diagnosis—it's a deeply personal and spiritual battle. And for Black Christian women, the war is often intensified by racial disparities, delayed detection, and fears around both treatment and faith.

The Stark Reality

While Black women are *less* likely to be diagnosed with breast cancer than white women, we are **42% more likely to die from it.** This isn't because our bodies are broken – it's because our systems are. This disparity stems from:

- Later diagnoses due to inconsistent access to screenings

- Higher rates of aggressive subtypes, such as triple-negative breast cancer

- Medical bias or dismissiveness toward our concerns

- Cultural silence around pain, fear, and health concerns

- Distrust in healthcare systems based on past injustices

- Spiritual guilt around illness (*"Did I not have enough faith?"*)

"I prayed the lump away instead of getting it checked. I was scared. And I didn't want to burden anyone."- J.H., 46, administrative assistant, South Carolina

But breast cancer thrives in silence. Early detection saves lives. Faith and science can work hand in hand to fight this disease.

Hormones, HRT, and Breast Cancer Risk

Hormones — particularly estrogen and progesterone — play a central role in both breast development and breast cancer risk. For women navigating perimenopause or menopause, hormone replacement therapy (HRT) is often suggested to ease symptoms like hot flashes, brain fog, and vaginal dryness.

But the type of HRT matters — a lot.

What the Research Shows:

- **Combined estrogen-progestagen therapies** (especially synthetic progestins) carry the highest breast cancer risk, particularly for estrogen receptor-positive tumors.

- **Estrogen-only therapies** also increase risk, but to a lesser extent.

- **Micronized (bioidentical) progesterone** appears to be less risky than synthetic progestins, though further research is still ongoing.

- **Vaginal estrogen** — used for dryness or urinary symptoms — has minimal systemic absorption and is currently not associated with increased breast cancer risk.

The duration of use matters, too:

- Risk increases can be seen even in the first 1–4 years of HRT.

- Longer use (5–14 years) significantly raises the chance of developing breast cancer.

- Discontinuing HRT generally lowers this risk over time.

This doesn't mean HRT is never appropriate—but it does mean a careful conversation with your doctor is crucial, especially if:

- You have a personal or family history of breast cancer

- You are BRCA-positive

- You're considering long-term or systemic hormone use

The Emotional Cost

Beyond the statistics, beyond the physical pain - there is a sacred truth: breast cancer affects the whole person and often brings emotional trauma.

- Fear of losing one's femininity or attractiveness:

    o *"Will I still feel like a woman after a mastectomy?"*- voice from a women's health circle in Houston

    o *"Will my spouse still be attracted to me?"* – voice from a women's health circle in Houston

- Anxiety around treatment side effects (like hair loss or mastectomy)

- Guilt or questioning faith

    o *"Why did God let this happen?"*- voice from a women's health circle in Houston

- Grief over body changes, fertility loss, or sexual intimacy struggles.

- "Why did this happen to me — did I miss something spiritually?"- voice from a women's health circle in Houston

Faith can be a refuge, but it can also feel like a battlefield.

- *"We are hard pressed on every side, but not crushed..."* – 2 Corinthians 4:8 (NIV)

- *"God is within her, she will not fall..."* – Psalm 46:5 (NIV)

Healing doesn't mean pretending you're okay. It means trusting God to walk with you, even through chemo, scans, and scars. Even in grief, there is grace. Your diagnosis is not your defeat. And your healing – body and spirit – is sacred ground.

Wholeness Strategy: Early Action and Spiritual Endurance

Medical & Hormonal Support

- Begin **mammograms annually by age 40**, earlier if you have a family history.

- Know your breast density—dense breasts can mask tumors on imaging.

- Ask about genetic testing (BRCA) if breast or ovarian cancer runs in your family.

- Discuss all hormone therapies with your provider:
  - If needed, vaginal estrogen is the lowest-risk option for symptom relief.
  - Micronized progesterone may offer a safer alternative than synthetic progestins.
  - If you've had breast cancer, systemic HRT is generally not recommended.

Nutritional Healing

- Prioritize anti-cancer nutrients:
  - **Cruciferous vegetables** (broccoli, cabbage)
  - **Berries** (rich in antioxidants) and **flaxseeds** (support hormone balance)
  - **Garlic, onions, turmeric, and green tea**
- Reduce inflammatory and hormone-disrupting foods:
  - Processed meats
  - Excess sugar
  - **Alcohol** – even small amounts can increase estrogen levels and raise breast cancer risk. Limiting or avoiding alcohol is one of the most impactful,

research-backed ways to reduce your risk.

  - o Highly processed foods

- Opt for:

  - o Herbal teas for hormone balance

  - o Omega-3 rich fish, like salmon or sardines

  - o Enjoying plant-based meals a few times a week

Lifestyle Shifts

- **Exercise regularly** to reduce recurrence risk and boost immunity.

- **Sleep and rest** deeply to support hormone balance and repair. It accelerates healing.

- **Talk it out**—join a support group, seek counseling, or confide in a trusted sister in Christ

Spiritual Anchors

- **Romans 8:28 (KJV):** *"All things work together for good to them that love God..."*

- **Isaiah 41:10 (NASB):** *"Do not fear, for I am with you... I will strengthen you."*

- **Journal Prompt:** "Where have I experienced God's comfort in the midst of my diagnosis?"

- **Prayer:** "Lord, walk with me through the shadows. Help me trust You with my healing, my identity, and my future. Meet me in the places that medicine can't reach. Strengthen me to walk this road in faith, not fear."

Voices of Victory

"I felt God's presence in every hospital room." – "Abby," 61, Florida
"Breast cancer took a part of my body—but it gave me a new sense of purpose." – A.W., 58, Georgia

"I thought breast cancer would end my life. Instead, it made me fight for it." – "Marie," 45, housewife, Connecticut

"My scars are sacred. They remind me I survived."- A.R., 67, retired teacher

---

This battle is real. But so is your strength. So is your support. And so is your God.

You are not your diagnosis. You are not broken. You are not alone. You are not less.

You are not less womanly, less worthy, or less anointed because of what your body has endured.

You are beloved.

And healing is yours to claim. And however your healing looks like – it is a holy, powerful thing.

Chapter 7: Sudden Storms – Stroke and the Fight to Restore Rhythm

---

"One minute I was fine. The next, I couldn't speak or move my arm."-
T.A., 51, behavioral therapist

"They said it was anxiety—but it turned out to be a mini-stroke."-

---

A **stroke** happens when the blood flow to part of your brain is suddenly blocked or reduced – either by a blood clot (ischemic stroke) or a burst blood vessel (hemorrhagic stroke). Without enough oxygen and nutrients, brain cells begin to die within minutes. That's why every second counts.

Stroke can lead to lasting damage – affecting your ability to speak, walk, remember, or even breathe. But not all strokes look the same. Some are dramatic. Others are quiet and easy to miss. Both are dangerous. Both require going straight to the hospital for life-saving intervention (like thrombolytic that dissolves blood clots).

Stroke doesn't always come with warning sirens. Sometimes, it's silent. Sudden. Disorienting. For

Black women, it's not just a medical emergency—it's a statistical reality.

We are **twice as likely** to experience a stroke as white women. And when we do, it often happens **earlier, more severely, and with worse outcomes**.

Why? The answer is layered—like everything else in our health journey. Stroke isn't just a vascular problem. It's also a hormonal, inflammatory, lifestyle, and spiritual crisis.

The Weight of the Numbers

Stroke is a leading cause of death and disability in Black women. Here's why it's particularly urgent:

- **Higher prevalence of hypertension**, the #1 stroke risk factor

- **Greater rates of insulin resistance, obesity, and high cholesterol**

- **Earlier onset of cardiovascular decline**— often starting before age 50

- **Delayed diagnosis** due to symptom misinterpretation (often dismissed as anxiety or stress)

- **Limited access** to stroke-preventive care or rapid intervention

And the consequences? Life-altering.

Paralysis. Slurred speech. Memory loss. Fatigue. Depression. Loss of independence. Fear.

Hormones, Blood Vessels, and the Perimenopause Storm

Stroke risk rises sharply after menopause—and not just because of age. It's because of hormonal shifts that directly affect your heart and blood vessels.

- **Estrogen** keeps blood vessels supple and helps regulate cholesterol and blood pressure. When it drops, arteries become stiffer, blood pressure rises, and plaque accumulates.

- **Progesterone** helps balance cortisol and maintain calm. Its decline may trigger sleep loss and stress sensitivity—both stroke risk factors.

- **Cortisol and insulin** climb with chronic stress and aging—fueling inflammation, high blood sugar, and blood clots.

This is why stroke prevention in women must include hormonal awareness—not just statins and aspirin.

The Hidden Signs – It's Not Always a Classic Stroke

We've been taught to look for FAST:

- **F**ace drooping
- **A**rm weakness
- **S**peech slurred
- **T**ime to call 911

But here's the problem: women—especially Black women—often present differently:

- Sudden fatigue or confusion
- Blurry vision or dizziness
- Nausea or trouble walking
- Headaches "like something exploded"
- Mood changes or brain fog
- Numbness without pain

And when we report it? We're often told:
"It's just stress." "You're probably dehydrated." "Try to rest."

We must learn to advocate, to insist, and to trust the signals our bodies are sending.

Faith and the Heart-Brain Connection

Scripture speaks of the heart often—but not just as an organ. As the seat of wisdom, emotion, and Spirit.

"Above all else, guard your heart, for everything you do flows from it."
—Proverbs 4:23 (NIV)

"You will keep him in perfect peace, whose mind is stayed on you."
—Isaiah 26:3 (KJV)

God created our minds and bodies to work in holy rhythm. But life's pressures—loss, grief, overwork, unresolved trauma—can interrupt that rhythm.

And when that rhythm breaks, it affects more than blood flow. It affects memory. Peace. Personality. Even identity.

But restoration is possible. And your healing is sacred.

Wholeness Strategy: Stroke Prevention and Recovery in Every Season

Medical & Hormonal Support

- **Routine checks** for blood pressure, cholesterol, and blood sugar—especially post-menopause.

- **Calcium heart scans** or carotid ultrasounds for women with family history or unexplained symptoms.

- **Ask about hormones**: If you're in perimenopause or menopause, ask how declining estrogen is affecting your vascular health.

- **If HRT is used**, favor transdermal estrogen with bioidentical progesterone under medical supervision (especially if stroke risk is elevated).

Nutritional Healing

- **Support vascular health** with:
  - Leafy greens, berries, fatty fish, flaxseed, garlic
  - Magnesium, potassium, and CoQ10 for blood pressure regulation

- **Avoid inflammatory foods**:
  - Processed meats, excess salt, trans fats, added sugars

- **Eat the rainbow**: Colorful fruits and veggies = brain and vessel protection

- **Hydrate wisely**: Dehydration thickens blood and raises stroke risk

Lifestyle Rhythms

- **Move daily**, not just for weight, but to boost circulation and lower inflammation

- **Prioritize deep sleep**, where your brain detoxes and your blood vessels reset

- **Release stress** through breathwork, therapy, worship, and joyful connection

- **Restoration, not just resistance**: Build rhythms of rest as a stroke prevention tool

Spiritual Anchors

- **Psalm 73:26 (NASB):** *"My heart and my flesh may fail, but God is the strength of my heart..."*

- **Isaiah 26:3 (KJV):** *"Thou wilt keep him in perfect peace, whose mind is stayed on thee..."*

- **James 1:5 (NIV):** *"If any of you lacks wisdom, you should ask God..."*

- **Journal Prompt:** "What burdens am I carrying that are breaking my heart in silence?"

- **Breath Prayer:** Inhale – *"Jesus, give me peace."* Exhale – *"Strengthen my heart."*

Voices of Renewal

"I found healing when I learned to say 'no' without guilt and 'yes' to myself."- C.R., 44, housewife

"God didn't ask me to die for the church. Jesus already did that."- "Nicole," 55, church administrator

---

Your heart is not just a pump—it's the wellspring of your spirit.
Your mind is not just a processor—it's the soil for your calling.

Stroke does not mean your story ends.

Let your healing begin not in fear, but in faith and informed love.
Let your healing be an act of worship.
Let your wholeness be your testimony.

You are the rhythm of your home, your church, and your generation.
Now it's time to restore your rhythm—for good.

Chapter 8: The Hidden Burden – Fibroids and the Quest for Relief

---

"I was bleeding so much, I had to carry extra clothes with me everywhere."- J.D., 45, registered nurse

"They told me fibroids were common and not to worry—but I couldn't go to work some days from the pain."- "Shirley," 37, South Carolina

---

Uterine fibroids – also called **leiomyomas** – are non-cancerous growths that develop in or around the uterus. They can be as small as a seed or as large as a melon, and often grown in clusters. While fibroids aren't usually life-threatening, they can cause heavy bleeding, pelvic pain, bloating, backaches, constipation, painful sex, and even infertility.

Many women don't even know they have fibroids until symptoms become unbearable, or they're told surgery is the only option. But there are more paths to healing than we're told.

For many Black Christian women, uterine fibroids feel like a secret struggle—common, yes, but far from harmless. They're often minimized by others and endured in silence, even as they disrupt our energy, fertility, and dignity.

But God sees every drop of blood, every night of pain, and every cry for relief.

The Disparity and the Delay

Fibroids are **three times more common** in Black women than in white women. We develop them earlier, grow them larger, and experience more severe symptoms.

By age 35, 60% of Black women have fibroids — compared to just 20–30% of white women. By age 50, that number rises to over 80%.

Yet many of us hear:
"It's just heavy periods."
"You'll feel better after menopause."
"You should just get a hysterectomy."

What we deserve to hear is the truth — and all of our options.

Hormonal Drivers and Bioidentical Hope

Fibroid growth is driven largely by hormones — especially estrogen and progesterone. This means, fibroids often appear or worsen during reproductive years and shrink after menopause. Black women often have earlier menarche, longer exposure to hormones, and genetic traits that increase sensitivity to hormonal changes.

Some treatments, like synthetic progestins in birth control, may alleviate symptoms short-term but can stimulate fibroid growth long-term. They also raise risks for LDL cholesterol increases, inflammation, bone loss, and blood clots.

In contrast, bioidentical hormone therapy (BHT) — which uses micronized progesterone and 17β-estradiol — shows promise as a safer, more effective alternative:

- Maintains cardiovascular neutrality

- Reduces fibroid volume modestly

- Carries lower clotting risk

- Offers better symptom control with fewer side effects

Though more studies are needed, bioidentical options provide hope — especially for women who want relief without surgery and without synthetic disruption to their natural rhythms.

More Than Physical: The Emotional and Spiritual Toll

Fibroids don't just affect the womb — they affect the whole woman.

- Lost pregnancies.

- Painful intimacy.

- Missed church services or career milestones.

- Silent grief over what could've been.

And beneath it all is the spiritual question: *"Why me?"*

But hear this:

- *"The LORD will sustain him on his sickbed; and restore him from his bed of illness."* – Psalm 41:3 (NASB)

- *"She is clothed with strength and dignity, and she laughs without fear of the future."* – Proverbs 31:25 (NLT)

You are not broken. You are beloved. And healing is still on the table.

Wholeness Strategy: Informed Choices, Inspired Faith

Medical & Hormonal Support

- Ask for a **pelvic ultrasound or MRI** to confirm fibroid size and location.

- Review **non-surgical options**:

    o **Bioidentical hormone therapy** (micronized progesterone + estradiol) –

may reduce symptoms and slow growth with fewer side effects.

- ○ **Uterine Fibroid Embolization (UFE)** – shrinks fibroids without removing the uterus.

- ○ **Uterine Fibroid Ablation** – aims to destroy fibroids directly using heat or other energy sources (such as radiofrequency energy).

- ○ **Focused Ultrasound (FUS)** – non-invasive, MRI-guided heat treatment.

- ○ **GnRH antagonists** (like Relugolix) – newer drugs that reduce fibroids without full menopause-like symptoms.

Avoid defaulting to hysterectomy unless it's truly needed — **you have choices.**

Nutritional Healing

- • Promote estrogen clearance and anti-fibroid support:

  - ○ **Flaxseed, cruciferous veggies**, beets, dandelion root

  - ○ **Green tea extract (EGCG)** – shown to reduce fibroid volume in studies

83

- Minimize inflammatory foods: sugar, dairy, red meat, processed snacks
- Hydrate deeply and consider **herbal allies** like vitex, turmeric, and milk thistle

Lifestyle Shifts

- Move to reduce inflammation: gentle cardio, strength training, stretching
- Detox daily: dry brushing, sweating, fiber, and sleep
- Reduce endocrine disruptors: switch to non-toxic beauty and cleaning products

Spiritual Anchors

- **Psalm 41:3 (NASB):** *"The LORD sustains him on his sickbed..."*
- **Proverbs 31:25 (NLT):** *"She laughs without fear of the future."*
- **2 Kings 20:5 (KJV):** *"I have heard thy prayer, I have seen thy tears: behold, I will heal thee."*
- **Journal Prompt:** "Where in my body or spirit do I need healing that I've been too afraid to ask for?"
- **Prayer:** "Lord, I give You my pain, my hormones, my hope. Heal not just my body—but my belief in what's possible."

Voices of Triumph

"I was told hysterectomy was my only choice. But I found a doctor who offered UFE and my life changed." – "Katrina," 35, New Jersey

"When I learned about bioidentical hormones, I felt empowered to choose what fit my body and my faith." – D.F., 40, Connecticut

"The bleeding didn't mean I was cursed — it meant I needed to advocate for my healing." – "Jill," 36, software engineer

---

You are not cursed. You are not weak. And you are not without options.

Your womb is not a battlefield — it is sacred space.

Let your healing begin with knowledge, compassion, and courage.

Chapter 9: Thyroid Troubles – Finding Rest and Regulation in a Tired Body

---

"I'm tired all the time — but my labs keep coming back 'normal.'" – L.F., 36, Florida

"I've gained weight, lost hair, and can't focus — but nobody seems to believe me." – M.G, 51, 5th grade teacher

---

There's a hidden battle happening in the bodies of many Black Christian women. It's not always loud or dramatic. It shows up as exhaustion, brain fog, cold hands, constipation, and weight that won't budge. It's a battle waged by a tiny butterfly-shaped gland called the thyroid.

And for far too many, this battle is missed, misdiagnosed, or misunderstood.

What Is the Thyroid and Why Does It Matter?

Your thyroid sits at the base of your neck and produces hormones that regulate metabolism, energy, temperature, mood, digestion, and menstrual cycles. When it's off — even slightly — everything feels off.

There are two main thyroid issues:

- **Hypothyroidism**: Underactive thyroid (too little hormone)

- **Hyperthyroidism**: Overactive thyroid (too much hormone)

Black women are often underdiagnosed with thyroid disorders, especially hypothyroidism, due to limited testing, racial bias, and generalized symptom dismissal.

And the symptoms? They're often mistaken for aging, depression, or stress.

Symptoms of Hypothyroidism Include:

- Fatigue, sluggishness, or constant tiredness

- Weight gain or difficulty losing weight

- Depression or mood swings

- Dry skin, thinning hair, or brittle nails

- Cold sensitivity

- Constipation

- Irregular periods or fertility issues

- Brain fog or memory trouble

- Puffy face or hoarseness

"It wasn't just in my head. It was in my hormones."- Katia, 33, choir member

The Hormonal Connection

Thyroid function doesn't exist in a vacuum — it's part of a hormonal symphony that includes:

- **Estrogen and progesterone**: Imbalances during perimenopause and menopause can disrupt thyroid hormone availability.

- **Cortisol**: Chronic stress suppresses thyroid hormone conversion, slowing metabolism and healing.

- **Insulin**: Thyroid dysfunction often travels with insulin resistance and PCOS, especially in women with abdominal weight gain.

And yet, many women are only tested for **TSH (thyroid-stimulating hormone)**—which gives an incomplete picture. You need to know your:

- **Free T3 and Free T4**: Active thyroid hormones

- **Reverse T3**: Inactive form (which can block function)

- **Thyroid antibodies (TPO, TGAb)**: Detect autoimmune thyroid disease like Hashimoto's

Don't settle for "normal." Seek *optimal*.

Faith and the Fatigue That Won't Quit

When your body is running on empty, but no one believes you, the exhaustion is more than physical — it's spiritual.

"I felt like I was failing at life, ministry, and motherhood. But really, I was just burned out—and no one saw it." - R.N., 53, women's ministry leader

But God sees. And He sustains.

- *"Come to me, all who are weary and burdened, and I will give you rest."* – Matthew 11:28 (NIV)

- *"He gives strength to the weary and increases the power of the weak."* – Isaiah 40:29 (NASB)

Rest isn't laziness. It's obedience — especially when your thyroid is crying out for help.

Wholeness Strategy: Reclaiming Energy with Wisdom

Medical & Hormonal Support

- Request comprehensive thyroid testing:
    - TSH, Free T3, Free T4
    - Reverse T3
    - TPO and TG antibodies

- If diagnosed:
    - **Levothyroxine (T4-only)** is standard, but many women do better with **combination therapy** (T4 + T3)

- Consider **natural desiccated thyroid** (e.g., Armour, NP Thyroid) with your provider's guidance

- Re-test regularly — especially during menopause, stress, or postpartum seasons

- Ask about **nutrient testing**: iron, ferritin, B12, selenium, zinc, and vitamin D are crucial for thyroid function

Nutritional Healing

- Support thyroid hormone production with:

  - **Iodine** (seaweed, iodized salt), **selenium** (Brazil nuts), **zinc** (pumpkin seeds), and **tyrosine** (eggs, chicken)

- Reduce goitrogens in excess: raw cruciferous veggies like cabbage and kale (cook them to lessen impact)

- Eliminate triggers: Gluten (if autoimmune thyroid), excessive sugar, and processed foods

- Try: Bone broth, turmeric, fermented foods (for gut support)

Lifestyle Shifts

- Prioritize sleep and recovery — thyroid healing requires deep rest

- Move gently but regularly — yoga, walking, stretching
- Support adrenal health with breathing, boundaries, and Sabbath rest

Spiritual Anchors

- **Matthew 11:28 (NIV):** *"Come to me... I will give you rest."*

- **Isaiah 40:29 (NASB):** *"He gives strength to the weary..."*

- **Hebrews 4:9-10 (NIV**): *"There remains... a Sabbath-rest for the people of God."*

- **Journal Prompt:** "Where have I been pushing through fatigue instead of surrendering it?"

- **Prayer:** "Lord, heal my thyroid and my pace. Help me live and serve from rest, not just routine."

Voices of Clarity

"Once I got the full thyroid panel, everything made sense." – R.B., 38, dietitian

"I stopped blaming myself for being tired. Now I'm healing—and learning to rest." – "Rachel," 43, mother of three

"God didn't ask me to hustle for my health. He asked

me to trust Him in it.”- Adrianna, 29, single mom and grad student

---

You are not lazy. You are not weak. And you are not imagining your symptoms.

Your tired body isn't broken — it's speaking.

Now it's time to listen with wisdom, respond with compassion, and reclaim the energy that is your birthright.

Chapter 10: Breathing Room – Asthma, Inflammation, and the Spirit of Breath

---

*"I feel like I'm suffocating —
physically and spiritually. Some
days, I can't even catch my breath
long enough to pray."* – "Imani," 31,
Connecticut

*"I was always told I had 'bad
allergies,' but now I've been in the ER
three times. Why didn't anyone take
me seriously?"* – "Keisha," 25,
lifeguard and praise dancer, Florida

For many Black Christian women, asthma isn't just a childhood diagnosis — it's a lifelong disruption. It shows up as wheezing during worship, breathlessness during choir rehearsal, or silent fear in the middle of the night. While asthma can affect anyone, Black women bear the greatest burden — **84% more likely to have asthma than Black men**.

And yet, the suffering is often minimized, delayed, or blamed on everything except what's actually going on inside the body, the home, and the environment.

It's time we tell the truth: asthma isn't just a medical condition — it's a justice issue. And it's a spiritual one too.

The Reality Behind the Wheeze

Nearly **1 in 9 Black adults lives with asthma**, and Black women lead those statistics. But the numbers don't stop at diagnosis:

- **Black individuals are nearly 3x more likely to die from asthma than white individuals**
- **Black children are 8x more likely to die from asthma than white children**
- **Emergency visits and hospitalizations for asthma are 4–6x more common in Black communities**

And yet, asthma deaths are mostly **preventable.**

So why are our people dying?

The answer: injustice in the air we breathe, the care we receive, and the communities we live in.

The Triggers We Don't Always See

Asthma can be triggered by many things — dust, smoke, mold, weather, exercise, and infections. But in Black communities, the causes go deeper:

- **Housing discrimination** means we're more likely to live in buildings with mold, pests, and poor ventilation.

- **Environmental racism** places Black neighborhoods near highways, factories, or landfills.

- **Healthcare gaps** mean we're less likely to be diagnosed early, given the right medications, or listened to by providers.

- **Chronic stress** from racism, economic strain, or over-functioning in faith spaces increases inflammation and weakens immunity.

This isn't about personal failure — it's about systems that choke our breath before we even recognize the danger.

Hormone–Asthma Connection: When Hormones Disrupt the Breath

"I noticed my asthma got worse right before my period, but no one ever told me hormones could affect my lungs." – "Antoinette," 36, waiter

"My breathing changed after menopause — tightness, wheezing, even night flare-ups. I thought it was just anxiety." – T.C., 63, grandmother and church health volunteer

For Black women, asthma is more than a respiratory issue — it's a hormonal issue too.

Studies show that estrogen, progesterone, and cortisol — the very hormones that shift during menstruation, pregnancy, and menopause—directly affect asthma symptoms and airway inflammation. And these shifts tend to hit Black women earlier, more severely, and with fewer treatment options.

Let's break it down:

- **Estrogen**: Can be both protective and inflammatory. During perimenopause or hormone imbalance, unstable estrogen may increase airway hyperreactivity.

- **Progesterone**: Low progesterone levels (especially common in PMS, perimenopause, and PCOS) can contribute to increased inflammation and bronchial sensitivity.

- **Cortisol**: The body's stress hormone. Chronic elevation — common in overextended, overburdened Black women — can trigger or worsen asthma symptoms through immune dysregulation.

- **Menstrual Cycle Effects**: Many women experience **perimenstrual asthma** (PMA), where symptoms worsen just before or during their cycle due to hormonal fluctuations.

- **Menopause**: Asthma prevalence **increases in postmenopausal women**, often coinciding with a drop in estrogen and an uptick in sleep disturbances, weight gain, and inflammation.

These hormonal shifts can lead to more frequent flares, medication resistance, and even nighttime attacks. Yet too many women are told, "It's just stress," or worse, "It's in your head."

It's not in your head. It's in your hormones, your history, and your environment. And you deserve answers that acknowledge all of you—not just your lungs.

Breath and Spirit: A Sacred Connection

In Scripture, breath isn't just biology — it's divine.

"Then the LORD God formed man of dust from the ground and breathed into his nostrils the breath of life..."
—Genesis 2:7 (NASB)

"He Himself gives to all people life and breath and all things."
—Acts 17:25 (NASB)

"Let everything that has breath praise the LORD."
—Psalm 150:6 (KJV)

Breath is holy. It is how we worship, live, and commune with God. So, when asthma threatens our breath, it strikes at the core of our worship and wellbeing.

Wholeness Strategy: Restoring the Breath God Gave You

Medical & Hormonal Support

- **Get proper testing**: If you struggle with chronic coughing, wheezing, or breathlessness, ask for a spirometry or peak flow test — not just allergy meds.

- **Use inhalers regularly**, not just when symptoms flare.

- **Track hormonal patterns**: Asthma may worsen around menstruation, pregnancy, or menopause. Estrogen and progesterone shifts affect inflammation and airway sensitivity.

- **Monitor for comorbidities**: Thyroid dysfunction, insulin resistance, and sleep apnea can worsen respiratory issues.

Nutritional Healing

- **Anti-inflammatory nutrients**: Omega-3s (salmon, flaxseed), magnesium (leafy greens, almonds), and antioxidants (berries, turmeric).

- **Avoid triggers**: Limit dairy, processed foods, and artificial additives that may increase mucus and inflammation.

- **Stay hydrated** to thin mucus and support lung function.

- **Consider gut support**: Poor gut health can increase systemic inflammation and allergic responses.

Lifestyle Shifts

- **Purify your environment**:
    - Use air purifiers at home (especially in bedrooms).
    - Avoid scented candles or air fresheners.
    - Remove mold, dust, and synthetic cleaning agents.

- **Practice breathwork**: Try 4-7-8 breathing, box breathing, or gentle singing to improve lung capacity and calm the nervous system.

- **Honor Sabbath Rest**: Fatigue and overexertion can trigger attacks. Your rest is protection.

Spiritual Anchors

- **Genesis 2:7 (NASB):** *"God breathed into his nostrils the breath of life…"*

- **Acts 17:25 (NASB):** *"He gives to all people life and breath…"*

- **Isaiah 26:3 (KJV):** *"Thou wilt keep him in perfect peace…"*
- **Journal Prompt**: "Where in my life do I feel breathless — not just physically, but spiritually? What is suffocating my peace?"

- **Prayer**: "Breath of God, breathe peace into my lungs, my spirit, and my space. Clear away every weight that steals my breath. Remind me that my breath is sacred — and so is my healing."

Voices of Freedom

"I used to think my asthma was punishment — until I realized it was a call to slow down and breathe with God." – E.N., 52, 8th grade teacher, New Jersey

"I got serious about my health after missing choir rehearsal for the third time. Now I treat my lungs like they're part of my calling." – M.L., 32, Human Resource Manager

"My inhaler is always in my purse — and so is my peppermint oil and Scripture card. I came to praise, not to wheeze." – V.T., 48, choir member

---

You Are Not a Burden. You Are Beloved.

Asthma may try to silence your breath — but your worship can't be stopped. You are not weak for needing help. You are wise for seeking healing. Your body is not broken — it is sacred space. And your breath is a gift from the very mouth of God.

Let's protect it. Let's honor it. Let's breathe — on purpose, in faith, and in freedom.

Chapter 11: Mind Matters – Anxiety, Depression, and the Battle for Peace

---

"I smile on Sunday, but cry in secret the rest of the week." – "Joycelin," 37, wife and mother of three

"I didn't know I was depressed. I just thought I wasn't praying hard enough." – "Maghalie," 34, wife and one year postpartum

---

For many Black Christian women, mental health isn't just about stress—it's about silence. It's about carrying the weight of being everything to everyone while feeling like you're falling apart inside.

"I'm always the strong one. But when I needed someone, no one checked in." – shared testimony from a virtual prayer group

"I serve, I give, I show up – but sometimes I wonder if anyone would notice if I disappeared." – shared testimony from a virtual prayer group

These aren't just passing thoughts – they're cries from the soul. In psychological terms, they reflect a lack of *mattering* – the fundamental human need to feel significant to others. Research indicates that when individuals feel they don't matter, they're more susceptible to depression, anxiety, and even suicidal thoughts.

We've been taught to "cast our cares" and "just trust God." But when depression lingers and anxiety steals your breath, faith doesn't mean pretending it doesn't exist.

Faith means facing it — with truth, support, and sacred compassion.

The Hidden Toll of Mental Health

Black women experience higher rates of depressive symptoms, chronic anxiety, and PTSD, but are less likely to be diagnosed or treated. We're expected to be strong, resilient, prayerful, and composed. The church, while a source of strength, can sometimes inadvertently contribute to this burden by emphasizing service over self-care.

And when we do ask for help? We're often told:

- "You're too blessed to be depressed."

- "Just pray it away."

- "Black women don't need therapy."

But the truth is — we do.

Because mental health is part of our whole health. And the brain, like the heart or liver, deserves healing too.

"Are not five sparrows sold for two pennies? Yet not one of them is forgotten by God."
—Luke 12:6 (NIV)

You are seen. You are valued. You matter.

Hormones and Mental Health

Anxiety and depression often increase during:

- Premenstrual phases (PMS, PMDD)

- Pregnancy and postpartum

- Perimenopause and menopause

Why? Because estrogen, progesterone, and cortisol all affect neurotransmitters like serotonin, dopamine, and GABA, which regulate mood, sleep, and energy.

Low progesterone can trigger anxiety.
Estrogen fluctuations can worsen irritability.
Chronic stress raises cortisol, which dampens joy and increases fear.

It's not all in your head — it's in your hormones too.

Symptoms to Pay Attention To:

- Persistent sadness or tearfulness

- Loss of interest in things once enjoyed

- Fatigue, brain fog, or sleep disturbances

- Panic attacks, tight chest, or racing heart

- Changes in appetite or weight

- Feelings of worthlessness, shame, or spiritual disconnection

- Thoughts of hurting yourself

"I was doing all the 'right things' spiritually — but emotionally, I was drowning." – "Beverly," 52, business owner

Faith and the Fog

Mental illness doesn't mean spiritual failure. It means you're human.

Elijah — God's powerful prophet — once prayed to die (1 Kings 19:4).
David cried through sleepless nights (Psalm 6).
Even Jesus wept under the weight of sorrow (John 11:35).

Your sadness is seen. Your struggle is not a sin.

- *"The LORD is close to the brokenhearted and saves those who are crushed in spirit." –* Psalm 34:18 (NIV)

- *"Cast all your anxiety on Him, because He cares for you." –* 1 Peter 5:7 (NASB)

Wholeness Strategy: Restoring Mind and Mood

Medical & Hormonal Support

- Ask your provider for:

  - **Thyroid panel, vitamin D, B12, iron, and sex hormones** — all impact mood

- Consider:
  - **Bioidentical progesterone** (especially in perimenopause)
  - **SSRIs or SNRIs** if needed — medication is not a lack of faith, it's a form of grace
  - **Therapy** — especially faith-informed or culturally competent therapists

Nutritional Healing

- Support neurotransmitters with:
  - **Omega-3s** (fatty fish, flaxseed, walnuts)
  - **Magnesium-rich foods** (dark chocolate, leafy greens, almonds)
  - **Protein** (chicken, eggs, legumes) to support dopamine and serotonin
- Limit: Sugar, caffeine, alcohol, ultra-processed foods

Lifestyle Shifts

- **Move to improve mood**: just 20–30 minutes of walking, stretching, or dancing can elevate serotonin
- **Sunlight and sleep** are both antidepressants — get both daily if possible

- Practice **grounding techniques**: deep breathing, Scripture meditation, journaling
- Connect with nature/God's creation
- Connect with others: Reach out for friendships and other relationships that are supportive, uplifting, and edifying

Spiritual Anchors

- **1 Peter 5:7 (NASB):** *"Cast all your anxiety on Him..."*
- **Philippians 4:6–7 (NIV):** *"Do not be anxious... and the peace of God... will guard your hearts and minds."*
- **Isaiah 26:3 (KJV):** *"Thou wilt keep him in perfect peace, whose mind is stayed on thee..."*
- **Journal Prompt:** "What fear or sadness am I hiding behind strength?"
- **Prayer:** "God of peace, meet me in the fog. Clear my mind, calm my heart, and remind me I'm never alone — even here."

Voices of Light

"Therapy and prayer saved my life. Both were gifts from God." – A.G., 64, Bible study leader

"I no longer see my anxiety as weakness. It's a signal

that I need rest — and I'm allowed to rest." – R.S., 39,
hair stylist

*"Depression didn't end my faith. It deepened it.
Because God met me in the dark."* – "Renee," 44,
North Carolina

Your mind matters. Your peace matters. Your emotional well-being matters to God.

You're not broken. You're not too much. You're not "just dramatic."

You are deeply loved, and your healing—mental, emotional, hormonal, and spiritual—is on the heart of your Heavenly Father.

Chapter 12: Chronic Pain and Inflammation – When the Body Speaks Through Suffering

"Every day, something hurts. And no one seems to believe how bad it is."
– "Abigail," 57, police officer

"I've prayed, I've pushed through, I've smiled through the pain—but I'm tired of pretending I'm okay." –
"Patricia," 63, retired Army Veteran

Chronic pain is a silent scream many Black Christian women live with daily. It's not just about one diagnosis — it's about years of symptoms, doctor visits, and dismissals. It's fatigue that doesn't lift, joints that ache without reason, and inflammation that simmers below the surface, often ignored.

For some, it shows up as an autoimmune disease. For others, fibromyalgia, arthritis, or unexplained back and muscle pain.

And too often, we're told to just *"lose weight," "rest more,"* or worse — *"it's all in your head."*

But your pain is not imagined. It's real. And it matters.

The Root of Inflammation

Inflammation is the body's natural response to injury or infection. But when it becomes chronic, it begins to harm instead of heal. It's a root cause behind many conditions Black women face disproportionately:

- **Lupus**

- **Rheumatoid arthritis**

- **Fibromyalgia**

- **Diabetes**

- **Obesity**

- **Heart disease**

- **Endometriosis**

- **PCOS**

Hormonal changes, especially during perimenopause and menopause, can worsen inflammation, triggering or amplifying these diseases. So can chronic stress, poor sleep, processed foods, and gut imbalances.

And yet, we often push through, downplay, or spiritualize our pain without ever addressing the root.

"I kept serving at church even though my joints were screaming. I thought quitting would make me selfish." – "Ms. Lee," 68, church greeter

God never asked us to suffer silently for the sake of service.

The Intersection of Pain and Faith

Pain can shake your confidence. It can make you feel broken or even punished. But Scripture reminds us that pain does not diminish your value or God's presence.

- *"The righteous person may have many troubles, but the LORD delivers him from them all."* – Psalm 34:19 (NIV)

- *"My grace is sufficient for you, for my power is made perfect in weakness."* – 2 Corinthians 12:9 (NASB)

- *"He was despised... a man of sorrows, acquainted with grief."* – Isaiah 53:3 (KJV)

Your Savior knows what suffering feels like. And He meets you in yours — not with shame, but with compassion.

Wholeness Strategy: Managing Pain with Purpose

Medical & Hormonal Support

- Request labs and evaluations to uncover root causes:
    - **Inflammation markers:** CRP, ESR, ANA panel
    - **Thyroid and sex hormone levels**
    - **Nutrient status:** vitamin D, B12, magnesium

- Consider advanced testing with a **functional medicine provider**:
  - **Comprehensive stool analysis** (e.g., GI-MAP or GI360) to assess gut inflammation, pathogens, and microbiome balance — key contributors to systemic inflammation
- Don't ignore symptoms that persist:
  - **Fatigue, joint pain, skin rashes, dry eyes, swelling, muscle weakness**
- Treatment considerations:
  - **Bioidentical hormone therapy** to stabilize hormone-driven inflammation
  - **BPC-157**: a synthetic peptide shown to reduce inflammation, promote tissue repair, regulate nitric oxide, and aid in connective tissue healing. It may help relieve musculoskeletal, gastrointestinal, and nerve-related chronic pain without toxicity.
  - **Microdosing GLP-1 agonists** (e.g., semaglutide): Small, individualized doses may reduce inflammation, oxidative stress, and cytokine levels (IL-6, TNF-α), offering potential pain and neuroprotective benefits. Microdosing

may also enhance tolerability and affordability for long-term use.

- If you are living with **obesity or excess weight**, know this: even modest weight loss (5-10% of your body weight) can significantly reduce inflammation, improve mobility (movement), and ease joint pressure.

- Don't be afraid to seek second opinions or explore emerging therapies under medical supervision.

Nutritional Healing

- Eat to calm inflammation:

  o **Omega-3s** (salmon, flaxseed oil)

  o **Turmeric, ginger, berries, leafy greens, olive oil**

  o **Bone broth, chia seeds, avocados**

- Avoid inflammation triggers:

  o Sugar, refined flour, processed meat, dairy (if sensitive)

- Experiment with an **elimination diet** (guided by a nutritionist or registered dietitian) to identify personal triggers

Lifestyle Shifts

- **Gentle, but regular, movement** improves circulation, reduces pain, and can even support weight loss.

  - Aim for 15-30 minutes a day.

  - Choose what your body can do joyfully: stretching, tai chi, swimming, dancing, or even chair-based workouts.

- **Epsom salt baths, massage, heat therapy** for daily relief

- Improve gut health — a key regulator of immune balance and inflammation

- Prioritize restorative sleep and stress reduction — because burnout inflames everything

Spiritual Anchors

- **Psalm 34:19 (NIV):** *"The LORD delivers him from them all."*

- **2 Corinthians 12:9 (NASB):** *"My power is made perfect in weakness."*

- **Isaiah 53:3 (KJV):** *"A man of sorrows... acquainted with grief."*

- **Journal Prompt:** "Where has pain become my identity—and what would it look like to let God redefine me?"

- **Prayer:** "Lord, I'm weary. I ask for healing in my body, strength in my spirit, and rest in my soul. Show me how to live with hope — even in the midst of the ache."

Voices of Endurance

"When I stopped hiding my pain and asked for help, God sent healing through both medicine and ministry." – C.P., 52, pastor's wife

"My inflammation didn't make me less holy — it made me more humble, more aware of my need for God." – "Yamile," 47, wife and teacher of 2nd graders

"I still have hard days—but I don't carry them alone anymore." - testimony from a virtual prayer group

---

You are not your pain. You are not lazy, dramatic, or defeated.

Your suffering matters. But it does not define you.

Let your body speak — but let wisdom, grace, and faith guide the healing.

Chapter 13: PCOS, Fertility, and the Desire to Be Whole

"I kept wondering what was wrong with me — irregular cycles, acne, weight gain, and no answers."-
"Candace," 32, store manager, Connecticut

"Every baby shower felt like a reminder that my womb was still waiting."- S.L., 38, Georgia

"The doctor said to lose weight, but didn't explain why my body was changing so fast or why my period disappeared."- K.K., 49, Florida

---

For many Black Christian women, **PCOS (Polycystic Ovary Syndrome)** feels like a maze without a map. It's not just about hormones — it's about identity, womanhood, and hope.

You're tired of being dismissed. Tired of being told it's your fault. Tired of the shame that creeps in every time your body doesn't do what it was "supposed" to do.

This is more than a medical condition. It's an emotional storm, a spiritual question, and a battle for wholeness.

And yet—PCOS is also an invitation. An invitation to understand your body, to advocate for your healing, and to believe that even in imbalance, you are not broken.

You are not behind. You are not less than. You are not forgotten.

What Is PCOS?

PCOS is a hormonal disorder that affects **1 in 10 women**, though the rates may be even higher in Black women. It involves:

- **Irregular or absent ovulation**
- **Excess androgen (male hormone) levels**
- **Ovarian cysts** (small fluid-filled sacs on the ovaries)

But beyond the ovaries, PCOS affects **the whole endocrine system**, often leading to:

- **Insulin resistance**
- **Weight gain (especially abdominal)**
- **Acne and excess hair**
- **Thinning scalp hair**
- **Anxiety or depression**

- **Infertility or irregular cycles**

PCOS isn't your fault. It isn't a punishment. And it's not the end of your hope.

Hormones and the PCOS Puzzle

PCOS is marked by disrupted communication between your brain, ovaries, and hormones. Key factors include:

- **Insulin resistance**, even in women of normal weight

- Elevated **LH** (luteinizing hormone), which disrupts ovulation

- Elevated **testosterone** and other androgens

- Low or imbalanced **progesterone**

These hormonal imbalances are not just cosmetic—they affect fertility, metabolism, and mood. Left unaddressed, PCOS increases the risk for:

- Type 2 diabetes

- Heart disease

- High cholesterol

- Sleep apnea

- Anxiety and depression

And yet, many Black women go undiagnosed or misdiagnosed due to bias, lack of provider awareness, or being told to "just lose weight."

The Fertility Struggle

For many women with PCOS, the pain of irregular cycles and hormonal imbalance is compounded by the ache of delayed or disrupted fertility.

Maybe you've spent years trying to track your ovulation, only to be told your body isn't working "right." Maybe you've tried to celebrate others while secretly mourning your own empty womb. Maybe you've laid hands on your belly in prayer, month after month, hoping for a miracle.

PCOS can make ovulation inconsistent or absent, making conception more difficult — but difficult does not mean impossible. Many women with PCOS go on to have children with the right support, timing, and medical care.

But fertility is about more than a pregnancy test — it's about identity, womanhood, and legacy. And when those dreams feel delayed, the spiritual weight can feel heavy.

- *"Why not me, Lord?"*

- *"Did I do something wrong?"*

- *"Am I less of a woman because I haven't conceived?"*

These are holy questions. And they deserve holy answers.

God's love for you is not diminished by your reproductive struggles. His plan for your life includes your healing—whether through physical restoration, spiritual motherhood, or new expressions of fruitfulness.

- *"He gives the childless woman a family, making her a happy mother of children." –* Psalm 113:9 (NLT)

- *"For this child I prayed; and the LORD has granted me my petition which I asked of Him."* – 1 Samuel 1:27 (KJV)

- *"No good thing will He withhold from them that walk uprightly." –* Psalm 84:11 (NASB)

A Hopeful Option: NaProTechnology

For those seeking a faith-aligned approach to fertility, **NaProTechnology (Natural Procreative Technology)** offers a science-based, dignity-affirming method of identifying and treating the root causes of infertility — including PCOS.

Using tools like the **Creighton Model FertilityCare System**, NaPro works with your body's natural cycles to:

- Identify ovulation patterns

- Detect hormonal imbalances

- Support natural fertility through targeted treatments like bioidentical hormone support, ovulation assistance, or surgical correction if needed

Unlike many conventional fertility protocols, NaPro doesn't override your cycle—it restores it. And for many Christian women, it offers a way to pursue conception without compromising faith values.

"With NaPro, I finally understood my cycle. I didn't feel broken — I felt seen." – "Nay," 29, wife navigating fertility

Wholeness Strategy: Nourishing Hormones and Rebuilding Hope

Medical & Hormonal Support

- Ask your provider to check:

    o **Testosterone, DHEA-S, LH/FSH ratio**

    o **Fasting insulin, glucose, A1C**

    o **Thyroid panel** (to rule out other causes of irregular periods)

- Treatment options to consider:

    o **Bioidentical progesterone** (supports cycle regulation and emotional well-being)

    o **Inositol supplements** (especially Myo-Inositol) to improve insulin sensitivity and ovulation

- **Metformin** (used off-label to address insulin resistance and cycle regulation)

- **Ovulation support**: letrozole, clomid, or timed interventions (if pursuing pregnancy)

- Ask about **microdosing GLP-1 agonists** (like semaglutide) to reduce insulin resistance and weight safely, with minimal side effects

- Seek out a health professional trained in **NaProTechology**

Nutritional Healing

- Focus on balancing blood sugar and reducing inflammation:
  - High-fiber, low-glycemic veggies
  - Protein and healthy fats at every meal
  - Cinnamon, apple cider vinegar, and green tea

- Reduce or avoid:
  - Processed carbs, sugary snacks, dairy (if sensitive), and hormone-injected meats

- Support hormone metabolism:
  - Cruciferous vegetables, flaxseed, and liver-supportive foods

Lifestyle Shifts

- Strength training + gentle cardio improve insulin sensitivity and ovulation

- Prioritize stress management: cortisol worsens hormonal imbalance

- Consider **GI testing (GI-MAP, GI360)** with a functional provider — gut inflammation and dysbiosis are often present in PCOS

- Consider At-home Hormone tracking devices, like **Mira** that allow you to track your estrogen, progesterone, LH, and FSH at home to better inform you of your hormone cycle trend that you can then share with a functional provider or NaPro Specialist.

Spiritual Anchors

- **Psalm 113:9 (NLT):** *"He gives the childless woman a family..."*

- **1 Samuel 1:27 (KJV):** *"For this child I prayed..."*

- **Romans 15:13 (NASB):** *"May the God of hope fill you with all joy and peace..."*

- **Journal Prompt:** "Where have I believed the lie that my body is failing me? What does God say instead?"

- **Prayer:** "Lord, you formed me with purpose. Help me treat my body with care, not criticism. Renew my hope and restore balance in every system."

Voices of Hope

"I stopped fighting my body and started learning how to support it. Everything changed." – "Natasha," 31, dance teacher

"God answered my prayer for a child—but He also healed my heart before the pregnancy came." – L.M., 40, social worker, Florida

"Even if I never carry a child, I carry purpose. I am still whole." – "April," 43, Sunday school teacher

---

PCOS is not a sentence — it's an invitation. To reclaim your health. To walk in grace. To remember that your value is not tied to your cycle or your fertility.

God's timing is perfect. His healing is complete. And your story is not over.

Part II: Living the Healing

The Final Chapter: Standing in the Gap – Reclaiming Health as a Sacred Act

---

"I didn't know how much I was neglecting my health until it started breaking down." – "Serena," 56, office manager

"Now I see my body not as a burden — but as a temple. And that changes everything." – "Caroline," 44, virtual assistant

---

Black Christian women are at the crossroads of resilience and risk. We are the backbone of our churches, our families, and our communities — and yet, too often, we put our health last.

This book has journeyed through the top ailments affecting our bodies—hypertension, blood sugar battles, heart disease, breast cancer, fibroids, thyroid dysfunction, mental health, chronic pain, PCOS, and more. We've uncovered the hormonal, nutritional, emotional, and spiritual threads running through them all.

And what we've found is this:

Healing is not just possible — it's sacred.

The Health Gap is Real—But It's Not the Final Word

Systemic disparities in access, bias in diagnosis, lack of culturally competent care — all contribute to the health gap Black women face. But so do silence, shame, and survival mode.

When we delay appointments, downplay symptoms, or disconnect from our bodies, we participate in the very systems that harm us.

And yet — we are also the solution.

We are not only daughters of the King. We are also keepers of the temple.

- *"Do you not know that your body is a temple of the Holy Spirit...?"* – 1 Corinthians 6:19 (NASB)

- *"She is clothed with strength and dignity, and she laughs without fear of the future."* – Proverbs 31:25 (NLT)

- *"The wise woman builds her house..."* – Proverbs 14:1 (KJV)

Now it's time to build—our bodies, our boundaries, our health ministries, our support networks.

Closing the Gap – With Wisdom, Faith, and Action

To reclaim health as a sacred act, we must:

1. Reclaim Our Voice

- Speak up about symptoms — early and often

- Ask for comprehensive labs and second opinions

- Choose providers who listen and respect your faith, culture, and concerns

2. Reclaim Our Rhythm

- Make space for rest, recovery, and Sabbath

- Nourish yourself without guilt or comparison

- Respect hormonal shifts — not as weakness, but as wisdom to adjust

3. Reclaim Our Community

- Start or join women's health groups at your church

- Mentor younger women in understanding their cycles, moods, and minds

- Normalize therapy, functional testing, and both prayer *and* practical care

4. Reclaim Our Legacy

- Track your health history — so your daughters don't walk blind

- Pass down not just recipes, but remedies and resilience

- Tell the truth about what hurt — and how God healed

You Are the Bridge

You are the generation that can close the health gap. Not with perfection. But with prayer, knowledge, and daily faithfulness.

- Faithfulness to schedule the checkup.

- Faithfulness to rest when your body says "no more."

- Faithfulness to treat food as fuel, not as shame or comfort.

- Faithfulness to ask God, "What would wholeness look like for me?"

Your healing is not selfish. It's generational.

Your wellness is not indulgent. It's prophetic.

And your wholeness? It's holy.

Prayer of Release and Renewal

Father God, I release every lie I've believed about my body — every word that called me broken, lazy, or unworthy. I receive Your truth: that I am fearfully and wonderfully made. Teach me to care for this temple with grace, wisdom, and joy. Let my healing ripple through generations. In Jesus' name, amen.

Appendix

Appendix A: Kitchen as Sanctuary

Recipes and Food Rhythms for Blood Sugar Balance, Hormone Health, and Holy Nourishment

To the daughter of God who Cooks with Purpose,

Your kitchen is not just a place of preparation — it's a place of healing. This addendum offers simple, functional recipes rooted in whole foods, cultural wisdom, and hormonal support. Each dish is designed to help regulate blood sugar, ease inflammation, and bring peace back to your plate. These are not diet foods. They are *soul foods*, reimagined — with intention, Scripture, and grace.

Recipe Title Index

1. **Peaceful Start Smoothie** – For hormonal balance and gentle mornings
2. **Healing Lentil & Sweet Potato Stew** – For blood sugar stability and comfort
3. **Holy Temple Power Bowl** – For estrogen detox and gut balance
4. **Luteal Phase Craving Bites** – For hormone-friendly snacking and cycle syncing
5. **Herbal Calm Tea Blend** – For cortisol relief and sacred rest
6. **Redeemed Mac & Greens** – A low-sodium, plant-based soul food classic

7. **Anointed Air-Fried Chicken Bites** – Crispy without the crash
8. **Garlicky Shrimp & Cauliflower Grits** – Blood pressure support with Southern flair
9. **Sautéed SuperGreens with ACV** – Metabolic reset greens with bold flavor
10. **Sunday Sweet Potato & Berry Bake** – A warm anti-inflammatory breakfast
11. **Crispy Okra, Black-Eyed Pea & Avocado Bowl** – A PCOS-friendly twist on tradition
12. **Collard & Cabbage Cancer-Fighter Stir Fry** – Quick greens with healing power
13. **Haitian-Inspired Pumpkin Soup ("Soup Joumou")** – Hypertension-friendly
14. **Coconut-Curried Red Beans & Plantains** – Thyroid supportive
15. **Caribbean Pineapple & Ginger Smoothie** – Fibroid management

---

1. Peaceful Start Smoothie

A creamy, nourishing way to ease into the morning — calms cortisol, balances blood sugar, and supports hormone health.

Prep Time: 5 minutes
Servings: 1
Inspired By: Morning prayer and fiber-filled, cycle-supportive smoothies

Supports: Blood sugar regulation, insulin sensitivity, energy stabilization

Ingredients

- ½ avocado
- ½ frozen banana
- 1 scoop unsweetened plant-based protein powder*
- 1 tbsp chia or flaxseeds
- ½ cup spinach
- 1 tsp cinnamon
- 1 cup unsweetened almond milk (or water)

Sidenote: choose a protein powder that is 3rd party verified to avoid contamination with heavy metals

Instructions

1. Add all ingredients into a blender.
2. Blend until smooth and creamy. Add more liquid as needed.
3. Sip slowly and prayerfully — set the tone for your day.

Why It Works:

- Avocado + seeds = healthy fats + fiber for blood sugar balance
- Cinnamon = natural glucose stabilizer
- Protein = supports cortisol control and appetite regulation

"Early will I seek You." —Psalm 63:1 (KJV)

2. Healing Lentil & Sweet Potato Stew

A warm, grounding one-pot meal rich in fiber, iron, and anti-inflammatory ingredients.

Prep + Cook Time: 40 minutes

Servings: 4

Inspired By: Hearty stews and Sunday "pot blessings"

Supports: Insulin sensitivity, immune resilience, hormone stability

Ingredients

- 1 cup dry lentils (rinsed)
- 1 medium sweet potato, diced
- 1 chopped carrot
- 1 small onion, diced
- 2 cloves garlic, minced
- 1 tsp turmeric
- ½ tsp cumin
- 4 cups low-sodium vegetable broth (can substitute with beef/chicken broth)
- Optional: chopped kale or spinach

Instructions

1. Sauté onion and garlic in a pot with olive oil until fragrant.
2. Add lentils, sweet potato, carrot, broth, turmeric, and cumin. Bring to a boil.
3. Reduce heat and simmer for 30–35 minutes until tender. Add greens in the last 5 minutes.
4. Serve warm, alone or over brown rice.

Why It Works:

- Lentils + sweet potatoes = slow-digesting carbs + minerals
- Turmeric = inflammation and pain modulator

- Iron + fiber = supports menstruation and detox

"The Lord sustains them on their sickbed." —
Psalm 41:3 (NASB)

3. Holy Temple Power Bowl

A rainbow of nutrient-dense foods that help your body detox, refuel, and heal from the inside out.

Prep + Cook Time: 25 minutes
Servings: 2
Inspired By: Deconstructed "soul plates" reimagined with balance and grace
Supports: Estrogen metabolism, gut health, blood sugar regulation

Ingredients
- ½ cup cooked quinoa or wild rice
- ½ cup roasted Brussels sprouts or broccoli
- ½ cup shredded carrots
- ½ cup baked salmon or roasted chickpeas
- ¼ avocado, sliced
- Handful of leafy greens (e.g., arugula or spinach)
- 1 tbsp tahini + lemon dressing

Instructions
1. Assemble all cooked and raw ingredients in a large bowl.
2. Drizzle with tahini-lemon dressing.
3. Eat slowly, mindfully, and in gratitude.

Why It Works:

- Cruciferous veggies = detox estrogen and reduce fibroids
- Protein + fiber + fat = stable glucose and satisfied appetite
- Tahini = calcium and healthy fat for hormone support

"Present your bodies a living sacrifice." —Romans 12:1 (NASB)

4. Luteal Phase Craving Bites

Cycle-friendly energy bites for when sweet cravings hit before your period.

Prep Time: 15 minutes
Chill Time: 1 hour
Servings: 10–12 bites
Inspired By: No-bake cookies and PMS cravings
Supports: Luteal phase balance, magnesium, mood, and fullness

Ingredients
- 1 cup rolled oats
- ⅓ cup almond butter
- 1 tbsp unsweetened cocoa powder
- 2 tbsp ground flax or chia seeds
- 2 tbsp honey or maple syrup
- 1 tsp vanilla extract
- Pinch of sea salt

Instructions

1. Mix all ingredients in a bowl until well combined.
2. Roll into 1-inch balls and place on a plate.
3. Chill for 1 hour in the fridge before serving.

Why It Works:
- Magnesium + healthy fats = ease cramping and mood swings
- Cocoa = antioxidant-rich and serotonin-supportive
- Fiber = balances blood sugar during the hormonal dip

"There is a time... to be filled." —Ecclesiastes 3:1, paraphrased (NIV)

5. Herbal Calm Tea Blend

A warming, relaxing tea that supports stress recovery and prepares the body for restful sleep.

Prep Time: 5 minutes
Steep Time: 5–7 minutes
Servings: 1–2 cups
Inspired By: Southern sweet tea, reimagined for healing and calm
Supports: Cortisol balance, sleep, digestion, hormone regulation

Ingredients
- 1 part dried chamomile
- 1 part dried lemon balm or lavender
- 1 cinnamon stick (or pinch ground cinnamon)

- Optional: 1 tsp raw honey + 1 tsp apple cider vinegar

Instructions

1. Steep herbs and cinnamon in hot water for 5–7 minutes.
2. Add honey or ACV if desired. Sip slowly.

Why It Works:

- Chamomile + lemon balm = calms the nervous system
- Cinnamon = stabilizes blood sugar, supports digestion
- Honey + ACV = gut-friendly and soothing

"He gives His beloved sleep." —Psalm 127:2 (KJV)

6. Redeemed Mac & Greens

A creamy, dairy-free, whole-food version of baked mac and cheese with collard greens.

Supports: Estrogen detox, gut health, anti-inflammatory balance
Prep Time: 20 minutes
Cook Time: 30 minutes
Serves: 6–8 (potluck portion)

Ingredients:

- 1 box chickpea or whole wheat elbow pasta
- 1 tbsp olive oil
- 1 small onion, diced
- 2 cloves garlic
- 3 cups collard greens, chopped

- 1 cup unsweetened oat or almond milk
- 1 cup steamed butternut squash or cooked sweet potato
- ½ cup nutritional yeast
- 1 tbsp tahini or cashew butter
- 1 tsp smoked paprika
- Sea salt + pepper to taste

Instructions:

1. Cook pasta according to package; drain and set aside.
2. Sauté onion and garlic in olive oil until soft. Add greens; cook until wilted.
3. Blend squash, milk, nutritional yeast, tahini, paprika, salt, and pepper until smooth.
4. Combine all and bake in a casserole dish at 350°F for 15–20 minutes. Optional: Top with almond meal or whole-grain breadcrumbs.

"They broke bread in their homes and ate together with glad and sincere hearts." —Acts 2:46 (NIV)

7. Anointed Air-Fried Chicken Bites

A crispy, flavor-packed alternative to traditional fried chicken—without the inflammation.

Supports: Blood sugar control, low inflammatory load, family-friendly
Prep Time: 15 minutes
Cook Time: 20–25 minutes (air fryer or oven)
Serves: 6–8 (potluck portion)

Ingredients:

- 2 lbs boneless chicken thighs or breast, cut into chunks
- 1 cup almond flour (or crushed whole-grain crackers)
- 1 tbsp ground flaxseed (optional for crunch + fiber)
- 1 tsp paprika, ½ tsp garlic powder, ½ tsp onion powder
- Sea salt + pepper to taste
- 2 eggs (or dairy-free milk + 1 tbsp mustard for egg-free option)
- Olive oil spray or brush

Instructions:

1. Preheat air fryer to 375°F (or oven to 400°F).
2. Mix almond flour, flaxseed, and spices in one bowl.
3. Dip chicken pieces into egg, then into flour mixture to coat.
4. Place in air fryer basket (or on parchment-lined baking sheet). Spray lightly with oil.
5. Cook for 18–25 minutes, flipping halfway.

Serve with mustard-garlic Greek yogurt sauce or avocado ranch.

"Taste and see that the Lord is good." —Psalm 34:8 (KJV)

8. Garlicky Shrimp & Creamy Cauliflower Grits

A soul food makeover that's blood pressure-friendly and full of flavor—without added sodium.

Prep + Cook Time: 35–40 minutes

Servings: 4

Supports: Heart health, insulin sensitivity, hormone balance

Ingredients
For the Shrimp:
- 1 lb large shrimp, peeled and deveined
- 1 tablespoon olive oil
- 4 cloves garlic, minced
- 1 teaspoon smoked paprika
- ½ teaspoon black pepper
- ½ teaspoon onion powder
- Juice of ½ lemon
- 1 tablespoon chopped parsley (optional)

For the Cauliflower "Grits":
- 1 large head cauliflower (or 1 bag riced cauliflower)
- ¼ cup unsweetened almond milk or low-sodium vegetable broth
- 1 tablespoon olive oil or plant-based butter
- ¼ teaspoon garlic powder
- ¼ teaspoon black pepper
- 2 tablespoons nutritional yeast
- Optional: pinch of crushed red pepper flakes

Instructions
1. Steam cauliflower 6–8 minutes until fork-tender. (Microwave if using riced cauliflower.)
2. Season shrimp with paprika, black pepper, onion powder, and lemon juice. Let rest.

3. In a skillet, heat olive oil over medium. Add garlic and sauté for 1 minute.
4. Add shrimp and cook 2–3 minutes per side until pink and opaque. Remove from heat; top with parsley.
5. For grits: Blend steamed cauliflower, almond milk, olive oil, garlic powder, pepper, and nutritional yeast until creamy.
6. Assemble: Serve grits in a bowl and top with shrimp. Garnish with lemon zest or red pepper flakes.

Why It's Blood Pressure Friendly:
- Cauliflower = potassium-rich, low-carb grit substitute
- Nutritional yeast = cheesy flavor without sodium
- Garlic, lemon, and smoked paprika = bold taste without added salt

"He fills the hungry with good things." —Luke 1:53 (NIV)

9. Sautéed SuperGreens with Garlic, Apple Cider Vinegar & Olive Oil

A weeknight-friendly side dish that supports hormones, metabolism, and digestion.

Prep + Cook Time: 25 minutes
Servings: 4

Ideal For: Metabolic reset, hormone balance, weight stability

Ingredients

- 1 bunch collard greens (or mix with kale, mustard, or turnip greens), chopped
- 1 tablespoon extra virgin olive oil
- 3–4 cloves garlic, minced
- ¼ red onion, thinly sliced
- 1 tablespoon raw, unfiltered apple cider vinegar
- ½ teaspoon smoked paprika
- ¼ teaspoon crushed red pepper flakes (optional)
- ¼ teaspoon black pepper
- Sea salt to taste (optional)

Optional Add-Ins for Extra Nutrient Support:

- Sliced mushrooms (estrogen detox)
- Diced tomatoes (vitamin C + antioxidants)
- 1 tablespoon hemp or pumpkin seeds (zinc + plant protein)
- ¼ cup cooked lentils (fiber + insulin support)

Instructions

1. Wash and chop greens, removing thick stems.
2. In a large skillet, heat olive oil over medium. Sauté garlic and onion for 2–3 minutes.
3. Add greens and sauté 3–5 minutes until wilted but vibrant.
4. Add smoked paprika, black pepper, and red pepper flakes (if using).

5. Stir in apple cider vinegar; cook 1–2 more minutes.
6. Finish with a light pinch of sea salt if needed. Serve warm.

Why It Works:
- Greens = rich in magnesium, folate, and fiber
- Olive oil = supports hormone and heart health
- Garlic & vinegar = may improve blood sugar regulation and gut health
- Low sodium = protects blood pressure and reduces fluid retention

"Beloved, I pray that you may prosper in all things and be in health, just as your soul prospers." —3 John 1:2 (NKJV)

10. Sunday Sweet Potato & Berry Breakfast Bake

A warm, baked breakfast that feels like cobbler but works like medicine—for inflammation, gut health, and blood sugar control.

Prep + Cook Time: 40 minutes
Servings: 4
Inspired By: Sunday sweet potato pie + cobbler
Supports: Inflammation, insulin resistance, gut healing

Ingredients:
- 1 medium sweet potato, peeled and thinly sliced

- 1 cup fresh or frozen mixed berries (blueberries, blackberries, raspberries)
- 1 tablespoon ground flaxseed
- ½ teaspoon cinnamon
- ¼ teaspoon nutmeg
- ½ teaspoon vanilla extract
- 1 tablespoon coconut oil or olive oil
- 1 teaspoon raw honey or maple syrup (optional)
- 1 tablespoon chopped pecans or walnuts (optional)

Instructions:

1. Preheat oven to 375°F. Grease a small baking dish with coconut oil.
2. In a bowl, toss sweet potato slices with oil, flaxseed, cinnamon, nutmeg, and vanilla.
3. Layer sweet potatoes and berries in the dish. Drizzle with honey (if using).
4. Cover and bake for 30–35 minutes. Uncover for last 10 minutes to crisp.
5. Top with chopped nuts if desired.

Why It Works:

- Sweet potato = anti-inflammatory, blood-sugar-friendly complex carb
- Berries = antioxidants that support joint, heart, and brain health
- Flaxseed = gut-friendly fiber + omega-3s

"He gives you food in due season." —Psalm 145:15 (NIV)

11. Crispy Okra, Black-Eyed Pea & Avocado Bowl

A Southern remix for PCOS—crunchy, creamy, blood sugar-friendly, and hormone-supportive.

Prep + Cook Time: 30 minutes
Servings: 2–3
Inspired By: Fried okra, Hoppin' John, and Southern veggie plates
Supports: PCOS, insulin resistance, fiber intake, ovary support

Ingredients:

- 1 cup fresh or frozen okra, sliced
- 1 tablespoon olive oil
- 1 cup cooked black-eyed peas
- ¼ red onion, diced
- ½ ripe avocado, diced
- ½ cup cooked brown rice or farro
- 1 tablespoon apple cider vinegar + ½ tsp Dijon mustard
- Optional: sprinkle of cayenne or smoked paprika

Instructions:

1. In a skillet, sauté okra in olive oil until crisp (10–12 minutes).
2. In a bowl, combine black-eyed peas, red onion, avocado, and rice.
3. Add sautéed okra and toss with vinegar + mustard. Season to taste.

Why It Works for PCOS:

- Black-eyed peas + okra = high-fiber, hormone-regulating superstars
- Avocado = healthy fat that improves insulin sensitivity
- No frying, no added sugar, no dairy

"You will eat the fruit of your labor—blessings and prosperity will be yours." —Psalm 128:2 (NIV)

12. Collard & Cabbage Cancer-Fighter Stir Fry

A one-pan wonder inspired by grandma's greens—but quicker, lighter, and full of anti-cancer nutrients.

Prep + Cook Time: 25 minutes
Servings: 4
Inspired By: Collards, cabbage, and Sunday dinner greens
Supports: Breast and uterine cancer prevention, estrogen metabolism, detox pathways

Ingredients:
- 1 tablespoon avocado or olive oil
- 2 cloves garlic, minced
- 2 cups chopped collard greens
- 2 cups shredded green or purple cabbage
- ½ carrot, grated
- 1 tablespoon apple cider vinegar
- ½ teaspoon turmeric + black pepper
- Optional: 1 tablespoon hemp seeds or nutritional yeast for topping

Instructions:

1. Heat oil in a skillet. Sauté garlic for 1 minute.
2. Add greens, cabbage, and carrot. Stir-fry 5–8 minutes until just tender.
3. Add vinegar, turmeric, and pepper. Stir to combine and reduce heat.
4. Top with hemp seeds or nutritional yeast if desired.

Why It Works for Hormone-Sensitive Conditions:

- Collards + cabbage = cruciferous veggies that detox excess estrogen
- Turmeric + pepper = reduce cancer-related inflammation
- Quick cook = keeps nutrients intact

"Her lamp does not go out at night... she provides food for her household." —Proverbs 31:15,18 (NIV)

13. Haitian-Inspired Pumpkin Soup ("Soup Joumou") — Low-Sodium Version

A heart-healthy remix of a beloved Haitian classic traditionally eaten on Haitian Independence Day.

Targets: Hypertension (High Blood Pressure), heart health
Prep + Cook Time: 60 minutes
Servings: 6–8

Ingredients:

- 2 cups pumpkin or butternut squash puree (fresh or canned)

- 2 tbsp olive oil
- 1 medium onion, diced
- 2 garlic cloves, minced
- 2 carrots, chopped
- 2 celery stalks, diced
- 1 sweet potato, diced
- 6 cups low-sodium vegetable broth
- 1 tsp turmeric
- ½ tsp black pepper
- 1 tbsp fresh thyme
- 1 bay leaf
- 1 cup chopped cabbage or kale
- Juice of 1 lime
- Optional protein: shredded chicken breast or kidney beans

Instructions:

1. Heat olive oil in a pot. Sauté onion, garlic, carrots, celery until tender.
2. Add pumpkin puree, sweet potato, broth, turmeric, thyme, bay leaf, and pepper. Simmer for 30 minutes.
3. Add cabbage or kale. Cook 10 more minutes.
4. Stir in lime juice and protein (if using). Serve hot.

Why It Helps Hypertension:

- Low sodium, potassium-rich ingredients
- Turmeric = anti-inflammatory, supports vascular health
- High-fiber veggies = help regulate blood pressure naturally

"A joyful heart is good medicine." —Proverbs 17:22 (NIV)

14. Coconut-Curried Red Beans & Plantains

A thyroid-friendly dish packed with iodine, selenium, and healthy fats inspired by Caribbean flavors.

Targets: Thyroid Health, metabolism
Prep + Cook Time: 40 minutes
Servings: 4

Ingredients:
- 1 can low-sodium red kidney beans, drained
- 1 tbsp coconut oil
- 1 onion, chopped
- 2 cloves garlic, minced
- 1 red bell pepper, diced
- 1 cup coconut milk (unsweetened)
- 1 tbsp curry powder
- ½ tsp turmeric
- ¼ tsp cayenne pepper (optional)
- 2 ripe plantains, sliced
- Fresh cilantro or parsley garnish
- Serve over quinoa or brown rice (optional)

Instructions:
1. Heat coconut oil. Sauté onions, garlic, and bell pepper until tender.
2. Stir in curry, turmeric, and cayenne. Add beans and coconut milk; simmer 10 minutes.
3. Pan-fry or air-fry plantain slices until golden.

4. Serve beans topped with plantains and cilantro over quinoa or rice.

Why It Supports Thyroid:
- Coconut milk + oil = healthy fats aiding hormone production
- Beans = iodine and selenium sources essential for thyroid
- Turmeric + curry = anti-inflammatory and antioxidant-rich

"You satisfy my soul with rich food." —Psalm 63:5 (NIV)

15. Caribbean Pineapple & Ginger Smoothie

A refreshing, anti-inflammatory smoothie specially crafted to help manage fibroids through liver detox and hormone balancing nutrients.

Targets: Fibroids, hormone detoxification
Prep Time: 5–7 minutes
Servings: 2

Ingredients:
- 1 cup fresh pineapple chunks
- 1 tbsp fresh ginger root, peeled
- 2 tbsp ground flaxseed
- ½ cucumber, peeled
- 1 cup fresh spinach or kale
- 1 tbsp raw honey (optional)
- Juice of ½ lime
- 1 cup water or coconut water

- Ice cubes (optional)

Instructions:
1. Add ingredients to blender.
2. Blend until smooth and refreshing. Serve immediately.

Why It Benefits Fibroids:
- Pineapple (bromelain) = reduces inflammation, aids digestion
- Ginger = reduces inflammation and supports liver detox
- Flaxseed = fiber and lignans, promoting estrogen clearance
- Leafy greens = chlorophyll-rich detoxification

"I pray that you may prosper and be in good health."—3 John 1:2 (NKJV)

Nourishment Is Ministry

Dear Daughter of God,

These recipes are not just meals. They are ministries.

Each bite you prepare is an act of resistance against diet culture, disease, and generational silence.
Each nutrient you receive is a step toward restoring the temple God entrusted to you.
Each meal you share is a reflection of the early church — where food, faith, and fellowship brought healing to the soul and body.

Let this not be about perfection, but about presence.
Let your time in the kitchen be covered in prayer and patience.
And let your nourishment become part of your worship.

"So whether you eat or drink, or whatever you do, do it all for the glory of God." —1 Corinthians 10:31 (NASB)

You are worthy of wellness.
You are called to be whole.
And you are not alone on this journey.

May your kitchen become a sanctuary.
May your meals become sacred.
And may your health become a living testimony of grace.

With you in faith and healing,

Kaleena Fransois Henry

Appendix B: Evidence-Based Resources

Below is a curated list of evidence-based resources, tools, and treatments mentioned throughout the book. These references are meant to empower readers to have informed discussions with their healthcare providers and explore a holistic path to wellness.

Medical Tests & Assessments

- **Comprehensive Hormonal Panels**:

    o estrogen (E2), progesterone, testosterone, DHEA-S

    o LH, FSH, SHBG (Sex Hormone-Binding Globulin)

    o Cortisol (AM/PM saliva or blood), Reverse T3, Insulin, Fasting glucose

    o Vitamin D, B12, Ferritin, Zinc, Magnesium

- **Thyroid Function Testing**: TSH, Free T3, Free T4, Reverse T3, TPO, TGAb

- **Cardiovascular & Stroke Risk Markers**:

    o Blood pressure (home monitor + office readings)

    o Lipid Panel (LDL, HDL, Triglycerides)

    o Calcium heart score or carotid ultrasound

- Inflammation Markers: CRP (C-Reactive Protein), ESR, ANA Panel
- **Metabolic & Blood Sugar Tests**: A1C, fasting glucose, fasting insulin, HOMA-IR index (Insulin Resistance Score), Waist circumference (visceral fat assessment)
- **Asthma & Lung Function**:
  - Spirometry
  - Peak Flow Measurement
  - Allergy testing (IgE panel or skin testing)
  - Hormonal review for perimenstrual asthma or menopause-onset asthma
- **Neurological Health:**
  - Brain MRI or CT (post-stroke evaluation)
  - Sleep study (if sleep apnea is suspected)
  - Cognitive assessment (memory, speech, mood after stroke)
- **GI & Inflammation Panels**:
  - **Stool Analysis**: GI-MAP by Diagnostic Solutions; GI360 by Genova Diagnostics (gut health, microbiome balance)

- SIBO Breath Test (Small Intestinal Bacterial Overgrowth)

- Zonulin (leaky gut marker)

- Food sensitivity and gluten reactivity panels

Emerging & Alternative Therapies

- **Bioidentical Hormone Therapy:**

    - Micronized progesterone and estradiol (transdermal patches, troches, or creams)

    - Especially relevant for menopause, PCOS, perimenstrual asthma, fibroids, or African American women who have increased hormone receptor sensitivity

    - Use with caution and supervision if stroke risk is elevated.

- **NaProTechnology**: Faith-aligned fertility and reproductive care using Creighton Model

- **BPC-157:**

    - A peptide with anti-inflammatory, gut-healing, pain-reducing, and nerve-regenerating properties

    - May support tissue healing post-stroke or in chronic pain syndromes

- **GLP-1 Agonists (e.g., Semaglutide):**

- Microdosing strategies for metabolic and inflammatory support

- Potential neuroprotective effects in pain and metabolic recovery.

- Early clinical studies report improved nerve regeneration.

- **Low-Dose Naltrexone (LDN):**

  - Used off-label for autoimmune pain and inflammation

  - May support conditions like Lupus, fibromyalgia, or chronic fatigue

Nutritional & Lifestyle Tools

- **Continuous Glucose Monitors (CGMs):** Real-time blood sugar tracking (e.g., Dexcom, Libre)

- **At-Home Hormone Tracking devices,** like Miracare.com, monitors specific hormones like estrogen, progesterone, LH, and FSH in real-time. This can be used for various purposes, including fertility tracking, perimenopause monitoring, or understanding overall hormonal health.

- **Inositol Supplements:** Particularly Myo-Inositol for PCOS and insulin resistance

- **Therapeutic Eating Patterns:**

- Anti-inflammatory: rich in berries, leafy greens, turmeric, olive oil, fish

- Blood sugar balance: low-glycemic carbs, Protein + high-fiber at every meal

- Hormone-supportive nutrition: cruciferous vegetables, flaxseed, omega-3s, healthy fats

- Vascular protection: Magnesium (greens), CoQ10, potassium (sweet potato, banana)

- **Supplements to Consider:**

  - Omega-3s fatty acids (brain + heart support)

  - Magnesium glycinate or citrate (sleep, blood pressure, anxiety)

  - Vitamin D3, B12, Zinc, Iron, Selenium (based on labs)

  - Inositol (especially Myo-Inositol for PCOS, insulin resistance)

  - Flaxseed and DIM (Diindolylmethane) (estrogen balance) or Calcium-D-Glucarate (estrogen metabolism support)

- **Breath & Stress Tools:**

- 4-7-8 breathing for cortisol reduction, reduce anxiety, lower blood pressure, and gently slow nervous system:
  - Inhale through your nose for 4 seconds, Hold your breath for 7 seconds, and Exhale slowly through your mouth for 8 seconds
- Grounding: Prayer walks, praise dance, forest bathing
- Mindfulness journaling + Breath prayers ("I am seen... I matter")

- **Home & Environment Support:**
  - HEPA air purifiers (especially for asthma)
  - Mold removal, dust mitigation, non-toxic cleaning products
  - Low-sodium seasoning swaps, whole food pantry staples

Mental & Emotional Support

- **Faith-Integrated Therapy Resources**

- **Trauma-Informed & Culturally Competent Therapy**
  - Seek Black Christian therapists when possible

- o   Incorporate spiritual + emotional healing (lament, rest, truth-telling)

- **Journaling and Scripture Meditation**

  - o   Scripture meditation + breathwork

  - o   Journaling prompts aligned with healing themes

- **Mindfulness Practices**: Breathwork, silence, gratitude routines

- **Support Groups**: Especially those led through churches, health ministries, or online Christian communities

- **Key Concept: Mattering**

  - o   Recognizing the deep human need to feel seen, heard, and valued

  - o   Lack of mattering is linked to anxiety, depression, and emotional exhaustion

  - o   Healing begins when women are treated not just as patients – but as whole people

Appendix C: Scriptural References

Sacred Scriptures for Healing, Wholeness, and Hope

These passages are woven throughout the book to remind you that your healing journey is not just physical — it is deeply spiritual. These verses are organized by theme to support reflection, prayer, and application in your daily life.

Wholeness & The Body

- 1 Corinthians 6:19–20 (NASB): "Do you not know that your body is a temple of the Holy Spirit..."

- Romans 12:1 (NASB): "Present your bodies as a living and holy sacrifice..."

- Psalm 139:14 (KJV): "I praise you because I am fearfully and wonderfully made..."

- 1 Samuel 16:7 (NIV): "The Lord does not look at the things people look at... the Lord looks at the heart."

Breath, Asthma & Restoration

- Genesis 2:7 (NASB): "Then the Lord God formed man of dust...and breathed into his nostrils the breath of life..."

- Acts 17:25 (NASB): "He Himself gives to all people life and breath and all things."

- Psalm 150:6 (KJV): "Let everything that hath breath praise the Lord."
- Isaiah 26:3 (KJV): "Thou wilt keep him in perfect peace, whose mind is stayed on thee..."

Mental Health, Peace & Mattering

- 1 Peter 5:7 (NASB): "Cast all your anxiety on Him, because He cares for you."
- Philippians 4:6–7 (NIV): "Do not be anxious about anything... and the peace of God... will guard your hearts and minds..."
- Isaiah 26:3 (KJV): "Thou wilt keep him in perfect peace, whose mind is stayed on thee..."
- Luke 12:6 (NIV): "Are not five sparrows sold for two pennies? Yet not one of them is forgotten by God."
- Psalm 73:26 (NASB): "My flesh and my heart may fail, but God is the strength of my heart..."

Heart, Stroke & Vascular Healing

- Proverbs 4:23 (NIV): "Above all else, guard your heart, for everything you do flows from it."
- Isaiah 26:3 (KJV): "Thou wilt keep him in perfect peace..."

- James 1:5 (NIV): "If any of you lacks wisdom, you should ask God…"

- Psalm 73:26 (NASB): "My flesh and my heart may fail, but God is the strength of my heart…"

Healing & Restoration

- Psalm 41:3 (NASB): "The LORD will sustain him on his sickbed; and restore him from his bed of illness."

- 2 Kings 20:5 (KJV): "I have heard thy prayer, I have seen thy tears: behold, I will heal thee."

- 2 Corinthians 12:9 (NASB): "My grace is sufficient for you, for My power is made perfect in weakness."

- Psalm 34:19 (NIV): "The righteous person may have many troubles, but the LORD delivers him from them all."

- Psalm 147:3 (NASB): "He heals the brokenhearted and binds up their wounds."

- Psalm 145:15 (NIV): "You give them their food in due season."

- Proverbs 17:22 (NIV): "A joyful heart is good medicine."

- 3 John 1:2 (NKJV): "I pray that you may prosper and be in good health."

Food, Nourishment, & Wellness:

- 1 Corinthians 10:31 (NASB): "So whether you eat or drink, or whatever you do, do it all for the glory of God."
- Acts 2:46 (NIV): "They broke bread in their homes and ate together with glad and sincere hearts."
- Psalm 34:8 (KJV): "Taste and see that the LORD is good."
- Luke 1:53 (NIV): "He has filled the hungry with good things…"
- Psalm 128:2 (NIV): "You will eat the fruit of your labor; blessings and prosperity will be yours."
- Ecclesiastes 3:1 (NIV): "There is a time for everything, and a season for every activity under the heavens."
- Psalm 63:1 (KJV): "Early will I seek Thee…"
- Proverbs 14:1 (KJV): "The wise woman builds her house…"
- Psalm 127:2 (KJV): "He gives His beloved sleep."
- Psalm 63:5 (NIV): "You satisfy my soul with rich food."

Fertility, Calling & Purpose

- Psalm 113:9 (NLT): "He gives the childless woman a family, making her a happy mother of children."

- 1 Samuel 1:27 (KJV): "For this child I prayed; and the LORD hath given me my petition..."

- Psalm 84:11 (NASB): "No good thing does He withhold from those who walk uprightly."

Discipline, Food & Balance

- 1 Corinthians 10:31 (NASB): "Whether you eat or drink... do all to the glory of God."

- Galatians 5:22–23 (NIV): "The fruit of the Spirit is love, joy... self-control."

Rest, Renewal & Strength

- Matthew 11:28 (NIV): "Come to me, all who are weary and burdened, and I will give you rest."

- Isaiah 40:29 (NASB): "He gives strength to the weary and increases the power of the weak."

- Hebrews 4:9–10 (NIV): "There remains... a Sabbath-rest for the people of God."

Appendix D: Scientific & Medical References

A curated list of peer-reviewed studies, clinical guidelines, and scientific literature that informed the therapeutic, hormonal, and nutritional strategies in this book.

Hormone Health & Bioidentical Therapies

- Holtorf, K. (2009). The bioidentical hormone debate: Are bioidentical hormones safer or more efficacious than commonly used synthetic versions? *Postgraduate Medicine*, 121(1), 73–85. https://doi.org/10.3810/pgm.2009.01.1963

- Fournier, A., Berrino, F., & Clavel-Chapelon, F. (2005). Unequal risks for breast cancer associated with different hormone replacement therapies: Results from the E3N cohort study. *International Journal of Cancer*, 114(3), 448–454.

- Manson, J.E., et al. (2019). Breast cancer and hormone replacement therapy: An individual participant meta-analysis. *The Lancet.* https://pubmed.ncbi.nlm.nih.gov/31474332/

- Santoro, N., Roeca, C., Peters, B. A., & Neal-Perry, G. (2021). The menopause transition: Signs, symptoms, and management options. *The Journal of Clinical Endocrinology &*

Metabolism, 106(1), 1–15.
https://doi.org/10.1210/clinem/dgaa764

- North American Menopause Society (NAMS).
(2021). *Nutrition and menopause: What you
need to know*. Retrieved from
https://www.menopause.org

- Mayo Clinic. (2022). *Menopause diet: Best
foods for women in menopause*. Retrieved
from https://www.mayoclinic.org

- Office on Women's Health. (2021).
Menopause and your health. Retrieved from
https://www.womenshealth.gov

- National Institute on Aging (NIA). (2022).
Menopause: Tips for healthy living. Retrieved
from https://www.nia.nih.gov

- North American Menopause Society (NAMS).
(2023). *Hormone therapy: Benefits and risks*.
Retrieved from https://www.menopause.org

- American College of Obstetricians and
Gynecologists (ACOG). (2023). *Management
of menopause*. Retrieved from
https://www.acog.org

- Hormone Replacement Therapy and Breast
Cancer Risk: Comprehensive review (2023).
Retrieved from
https://pubmed.ncbi.nlm.nih.gov/31474332/

- Johns Hopkins Medicine. (2023). *Managing menopause symptoms*. Retrieved from https://www.hopkinsmedicine.org

- Food and Drug Administration (FDA). (2022). *Hormone replacement therapy: Benefits and risks*. Retrieved from https://www.fda.gov

- BlackDoctor.org. (n.d.). *The 7 deadliest diseases in the Black community*. Retrieved from https://blackdoctor.org/the-7-deadliest-diseases-for-blacks/

- Black Women's Health Disparities and Menopause. (2024). *Black Women and Perimenopause Care Report*. Retrieved from https://www.uchicagomedicine.org/forefront/womens-health-articles/2022/october/hormone-therapy-research-race-menopause

- Harvard T.H. Chan School of Public Health. (n.d.). *Nutrition and healthy aging*. Retrieved from https://www.hsph.harvard.edu

- Women's Health Concern. (2021). *Nutrition and lifestyle in menopause*. Retrieved from https://www.womens-health-concern.org

- Stute, P., et al. (2021). Treatment options for genitourinary syndrome of menopause: Hormone therapy and beyond. *Maturitas*, 144, 76–82.

Cardiometabolic Health & Stroke

- Kalinowski, P., et al. (2022). Benefits of microdosing GLP-1 Agonists like semaglutide in metabolic syndrome and inflammation. *Journal of Clinical Metabolism & Endocrinology.*

- Lobo, R. A. (2017). Metabolic syndrome, inflammation and cardiovascular risk in women: Therapeutic implications. *Climacteric*, 20(6), 473–478.

- CDC. (2023). Stroke facts. *Centers for Disease Control and Prevention.* https://www.cdc.gov/stroke/facts.htm

Asthma & Disparities in Black Communities

- Hearne, M., et al. (2023). Asthma disparities in Black Americans: A critical analysis of prevalence, causes, and health outcomes. *Journal of Asthma and Allergy*, 16, 89–105. https://www.ncbi.nlm.nih.gov/pmc/articles/PMC10640900/

- National Heart, Lung, and Blood Institute. (2021). *Asthma in the Black Community Fact Sheet.* https://www.nhlbi.nih.gov/files/publications/asthma_in_black_community_fact_sheet.pdf

- Zein, J. G., & Erzurum, S. C. (2015). Asthma is different in women. *Current Allergy and*

Asthma Reports, 15(6), 28.
https://doi.org/10.1007/s11882-015-0528-y

- Leynaert, B., Sunyer, J., Garcia-Esteban, R., et al. (2012). Gender differences in prevalence, diagnosis, and incidence of allergic and non-allergic asthma. *Thorax*, 67(7), 625–631. https://doi.org/10.1136/thoraxjnl-2011-201249

Mental Health, Mattering & Emotional Wellness

- Prilleltensky, I. (2023). Mattering: A critical concept for health and well-being. *International Journal of Wellbeing*, 13(1), 1–20. https://www.ncbi.nlm.nih.gov/pmc/articles/PMC9970286/

- Howard, L. M., Ehrlich, A. M., Gamlen, F., & Oram, S. (2019). Women's mental health: A clinical overview. *The Lancet Psychiatry*, 6(7), 587–596.

- Schmidt, P. J., et al. (2000). Estrogen replacement in perimenopause-related depression: A preliminary report. *American Journal of Obstetrics and Gynecology*, 183(2), 414–420.

- Geronimus, A. T., Hicken, M., Keene, D., & Bound, J. (2006). "Weathering" and age patterns of allostatic load scores among blacks and whites in the United States.

American Journal of Public Health, 96(5), 826–833.
https://doi.org/10.2105/AJPH.2004.060749

Chronic Pain, Peptides & Inflammation

- Chen, L., et al. (2024). Microdosing GLP-1 receptor agonists in metabolic inflammation. *Diabetes Care*.
https://pubmed.ncbi.nlm.nih.gov/30741689/

- Sikiric, P., et al. (2020). Therapeutic potential of BPC-157 in chronic pain and inflammatory disorders. *Current Pharmaceutical Design*, 26(7), 785–802.
https://pubmed.ncbi.nlm.nih.gov/34380875/

- Sikiric, P., et al. (2021). Therapeutic potential of BPC-157 in chronic pain and inflammation. *Frontiers in Pharmacology*.
https://pubmed.ncbi.nlm.nih.gov/34380875/

- Pizzorno, J. (2016). The Human Microbiome: An emerging key to health and disease. *Integrative Medicine: A Clinician's Journal*, 15(6), 8–14.

- Floryn Health. (2024). Clinical applications of microdosed semaglutide.
https://pmc.ncbi.nlm.nih.gov/articles/PMC10992717/

Obesity, Weight, and Metabolism

- CDC. (2021). Prevalence of obesity among adults and youth. https://www.cdc.gov/obesity/data/adult.html

- Ogden, C. L., Carroll, M. D., Fryar, C. D., & Flegal, K. M. (2015). Prevalence of obesity among adults and youth: United States, 2011–2014. *NCHS Data Brief*, no 219.

- Hall, K. D., & Guo, J. (2017). Obesity energetics: Body weight regulation and the effects of diet composition. *Gastroenterology*, 152(7), 1718–1727. https://doi.org/10.1053/j.gastro.2017.01.052

- Lean, M. E., et al. (2018). Primary care-led weight management for remission of type 2 diabetes (DiRECT): An open-label, cluster-randomised trial. *The Lancet*, 391(10120), 541–551. https://doi.org/10.1016/S0140-6736(1733102-1

Neurology & Stroke Recovery

- Mozaffarian, D., et al. (2015). Executive Summary: Heart disease and stroke statistics—2015 update. *Circulation*, 131(4), 434–441.

- American Stroke Association. (2022). *Life after stroke: Our guide to recovery*. https://www.stroke.org

- Benjamin, E. J., et al. (2019). Heart disease and stroke statistics—2019 update: A report from the American Heart Association. *Circulation*, 139(10), e56–e528. https://doi.org/10.1161/CIR.00000000000006 59

Women's Health & PCOS

- Legro, R. S., et al. (2013). Diagnosis and treatment of polycystic ovary syndrome: An Endocrine Society clinical practice guideline. *Journal of Clinical Endocrinology & Metabolism*, 98(12), 4565–4592.

- Hilgers, T. W. (2004). *The medical and surgical practice of NaProTechnology*. Omaha, NE: Pope Paul VI Institute Press.

- Taylor, R.N., et al. (2023). Comparative efficacy of bioidentical vs. synthetic hormones in fibroid treatment. *Journal of Women's Health*. https://pubmed.ncbi.nlm.nih.gov/31834160/

- Wise, L. A., & Laughlin-Tommaso, S. K. (2016). Epidemiology of uterine fibroids: From menarche to menopause. *Clinical Obstetrics and Gynecology*, 59(1), 2–24. https://doi.org/10.1097/GRF.00000000000001 64

Menstrual Cycle, Hormones & Insulin Sensitivity

- Valle-Rios, R., et al. (2023). Menstrual cycle phase modulates glucose metabolism and insulin sensitivity in healthy women: A systematic review. *Frontiers in Endocrinology*, 14, 1124691. https://doi.org/10.3389/fendo.2023.1124691

- Yeung, E. H., Zhang, C., Mumford, S. L., et al. (2010). Longitudinal study of insulin resistance and sex hormones across the menstrual cycle: The BioCycle Study. *The Journal of Clinical Endocrinology & Metabolism*, 95(12), 5435–5442. https://doi.org/10.1210/jc.2010-0904

- Sims, S. T., & Heather, A. K. (2018). Myths and methodologies: Reducing scientific design ambiguity in studies comparing sex and menstrual cycle effects. *Journal of Applied Physiology*, 125(6), 1985–1996. https://doi.org/10.1152/japplphysiol.00662.2018

- Shaikh, M. G., et al. (2020). Influence of the menstrual cycle on metabolic parameters: Implications for clinical care. *BMC Endocrine Disorders*, 20(1), 22. https://bmcendocrdisord.biomedcentral.com/articles/10.1186/s12902-020-00521-3

- Sims, S. T. (2016). *ROAR: How to Match Your Food and Fitness to Your Unique Female*

Physiology for Optimum Performance, Great Health, and a Strong, Lean Body for Life. Rodale Books.

Disparities in Black Women's Health

- Baird, D. D., et al. (2003). Uterine leiomyomata in black and white women: Clinical and epidemiologic determinants. *American Journal of Obstetrics and Gynecology*, 188(1), 100–107.

- Woods-Giscombé, C. L. (2010). Superwoman Schema: African American Women's Views on Stress, Strength, and Health. *Qualitative Health Research*, 20(5), 668–683.

- Woods-Giscombé, C. L., & Black, A. R. (2010). Mind-body interventions to reduce risk for health disparities related to stress and strength among African American women: The potential of mindfulness-based stress reduction, loving-kindness, and the NTU therapeutic framework. *Complementary Health Practice Review*, 15(3), 115–131. https://doi.org/10.1177/1533210110386776

- Breathett, K., et al. (2019). Health disparities in heart failure and other cardiovascular diseases in African Americans. *Circulation: Heart Failure*, 12(4), e005572.

Functional Foods, Hormonal Nutrition & Culinary Medicine

- Katz, D. L., & Meller, S. (2014). Can we say what diet is best for health? *Annual Review of Public Health*, 35, 83–103. https://doi.org/10.1146/annurev-publhealth-032013-182351

- Menke, A., Casagrande, S., Geiss, L., & Cowie, C. C. (2015). Prevalence of and trends in diabetes among adults in the United States, 1988–2012. *JAMA*, 314(10), 1021–1029. https://doi.org/10.1001/jama.2015.10029

- Barrea, L., Muscogiuri, G., Macchia, P. E., et al. (2020). Nutrition and women's hormones: The pivotal role of micronutrients in hormonal balance. *Nutrients*, 12(8), 2323. https://doi.org/10.3390/nu12082323

- Basu, A., Rhone, M., & Lyons, T. J. (2010). Berries: Emerging impact on cardiovascular health. *Nutrition Reviews*, 68(3), 168–177. https://doi.org/10.1111/j.1753-4887.2010.00273.x

- Wallace, T. C., & Slavin, M. (2016). Dietary fiber and gut health: An overview. *Nutrition*, 32(2), 171–176. https://doi.org/10.1016/j.nut.2015.09.008

- Bahadoran, Z., Mirmiran, P., & Azizi, F. (2013). Dietary polyphenols as potential nutraceuticals in management of diabetes: A review. *Journal of Diabetes and Metabolic Disorders*, 12(1), 43. https://doi.org/10.1186/2251-6581-12-43

- Dehghan, M., Mente, A., Zhang, X., et al. (2017). Associations of fats and carbohydrate intake with cardiovascular disease and mortality in 18 countries (PURE): A prospective cohort study. *The Lancet*, 390(10107), 2050–2062. https://doi.org/10.1016/S0140-6736(17)32252-3

- Appel, L. J., et al. (2006). Dietary approaches to prevent and treat hypertension: A scientific statement from the American Heart Association. *Hypertension*, 47(2), 296–308. https://doi.org/10.1161/01.HYP.0000202568.01167.B6

- Zimmermann, M. B. (2012). The effects of iodine deficiency in pregnancy and infancy. *Paediatric and Perinatal Epidemiology*, 26(Suppl 1), 108–117. https://doi.org/10.1111/j.1365-3016.2012.01275.x

- Barrea, L., et al. (2019). Nutrition and thyroid: Nutritional factors in thyroid diseases.

Nutrients, 11(9), 2214.
https://doi.org/10.3390/nu11092214

- Zhang, X., et al. (2016). Dietary isoflavones or lignans intake and uterine fibroids: A meta-analysis. *PLoS ONE*, 11(2), e0148522. https://doi.org/10.1371/journal.pone.0148522

- Rondanelli, M., et al. (2021). Bromelain: A review of its therapeutic applications. *Journal of Clinical Medicine*, 10(19), 4522. https://doi.org/10.3390/jcm10194522

- Mashhadi, N. S., et al. (2013). Anti-inflammatory and anti-oxidative effects of ginger in health and physical activity. *International Journal of Preventive Medicine*, 4(Suppl 1), S36–S42. https://pubmed.ncbi.nlm.nih.gov/23717767

- Pahlavani, N., et al. (2014). Nutritional aspects of turmeric (curcumin): Health benefits and risks. *Journal of Medicinal Food*, 17(10), 1106–1112. https://doi.org/10.1089/jmf.2013.3110

- Sealy-Jefferson, S., et al. (2020). Food deserts, neighborhood poverty, and African American women's health: Challenges and solutions. *Health Education & Behavior*, 47(4), 517–523. https://doi.org/10.1177/1090198119887768

From the Author: A Closing Word of Encouragement

Beloved Reader,

If you've made it to this page, I want to pause and simply say — thank you.

Thank you for choosing to invest in your healing.
Thank you for daring to believe that your body is worth understanding.
Thank you for showing up — scars, prayers, questions, and all.

This book was born out of a deep burden - and a holy calling.

As a Black Christian woman and healthcare profession, I've seen firsthand the silent storms our bodies endure. Hyperension. Diababes. Obesity. Fibroids. Stroke. Depression. Chronic pain. All disproportionately affecting us. All too often dismissed or misunderstood.

So this book was created with you in mind.

To shine a light on the top health challenges that impact Black women of faith,

To explore their root causes – not just symptoms, and to offer faith-filled, functional, and culturally grounded tools to pursue healing – not just physically, but hormonally, emotionally, and spiritually.

This book was never about perfection. It was always about permission.

Permission to listen to your body.
Permission to ask questions and seek answers.
Permission to be a woman of faith who also seeks medical help.
Permission to rest, to change, to grow.

You are not just a statistic. You are a sacred story.

Whether you are walking through diagnosis, recovery, motherhood, grief, or rebirth—know this: God is not distant from your health journey. He is intimately involved, gently guiding you toward wholeness in every chapter of your life.

And now, as you go forward, I leave you with this charge:

- Be a bridge—between what was and what could be.

- Be a voice—in the doctor's office, in your family, in your church.

- Be a light—for the women still waiting to hear, "You are not alone."

And as you take the next step, I urge you:

Do not walk alone.

Surround yourself with mentors who understand your struggle, believers who pray and pursue wellness with wisdom, and healthcare professionals who honor your voice, your values, and your unique path.

You deserve care that sees you wholly – body, mind, and spirit.

You are a temple. A teacher. A torchbearer.
You are beloved.

May your healing ripple through generations.
May your story rewrite someone else's silence.
And may your life testify: wholeness is possible—and it is holy.

With gratitude and grace,

Kaleena Fransois Henry

About the Author

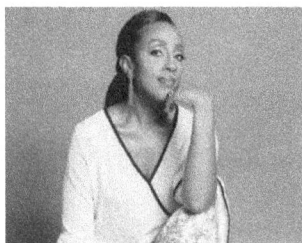

Kaleena François Henry, MCMSc, PA-C, is a board-certified Physician Assistant and Integrative Functional Nutrition Certified Practitioner with over 16 years of clinical experience specializing in endocrinology, metabolism, integrative functional medicine and women's health. Often known clinically as Kaleena François or PA François, her mission is to provide personalized, holistic care that blends complex medical experience with a passion for faith-centered, culturally sensitive wellness.

As founder of URENÜ LLC and Renewed Beginnings Holistic Health LLC, she empowers, women, especially Black Christian women, to reclaim their health through evidence-based nutrition, lifestyle coaching, and hormone harmony grounded in biblical truth. Kaleena also serves as an adjunct professor, guiding the next generation of healthcare providers with a focus on patient-centered, root-cause medicine.

Inspired by Hosea 4:6 — *"My people perish for lack of knowledge"* — Kaleena dedicates her professional life to education in all its facets. She believes firmly that *"tout pou bon Dieu"* (everything is for God) and that *"the secret of success is the consistency of purpose."* Through her integrative approach, which honors the sacredness of the body as God's temple, Kaleena advocates for healing that restores mind, body, and spirit.

Through her writing, coaching, and teaching, she invites women to walk confidently in wholeness, breaking cycles of silence and embracing their God-given vitality.

www.ingramcontent.com/pod-product-compliance
Lightning Source LLC
Chambersburg PA
CBHW050650270326
41927CB00012B/2965